Still Standing

Still Standing

JESS QUINN

WHAT I'VE LEARNT
FROM A LIFE
LIVED DIFFERENTLY

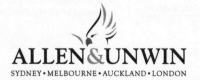

ALLEN&UNWIN
SYDNEY·MELBOURNE·AUCKLAND·LONDON

Allen & Unwin
Level 2, 10 College Hill, Freemans Bay
Auckland 1011, New Zealand
Phone: (64 9) 377 3800
Email: auckland@allenandunwin.com
Web: www.allenandunwin.co.nz

83 Alexander Street
Crows Nest NSW 2065, Australia
Phone: (61 2) 8425 0100

A catalogue record for this book is available from the
National Library of New Zealand.

ISBN 978 1 98854 729 9

Design by Kate Barraclough
Set in Adobe Caslon Pro
Printed in Australia by McPherson's Printing Group

1 3 5 7 9 10 8 6 4 2

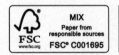

The paper in this book is FSC® certified.
FSC® promotes environmentally responsible,
socially beneficial and economically viable
management of the world's forests.

To Mum, Dad, Abby and Sophie-Rose
— you are the reason I'm still standing.

Contents

' One day you will tell your story of how you overcame, and it will be someone else's survival guide. **'**

I LOVE THIS SAYING. I don't actually know who said it first — it wasn't me — but it's become my motto. It's how I plan to live my life.

You're about to read my story. Sharing it has always felt right to me and, although it hasn't always been an easy way to live, it's always felt like my calling.

At times, this story has been hard to write, but I stand by it — every raw and honest word — because it's mine. I want to share it with you because I want you to know about the things I have overcome, and the things I hope to overcome. I want you to see what's possible. I want my best days, my proudest achievements, to be an example of why hope always has a place. I want my darkest days to be the glimmer of hope you might need to push through your darkest times.

I believe in the power of storytelling. We all hold stories that need to be shared. One thing I have learnt through sharing my story is that you truly never know who might need to hear *yours*. The darkness in your life may be the light someone else needs to get through. It may be the common ground a stranger needs to find sure footing. And the glowing moments? They might be just the inspiration someone needs to keep going.

Life is about more than just us. The world we live in, the people we share it with, and the time that we're here — it's all part of a collection of stories. At every moment, every single one of our personal stories is alive and unfolding, pulling from those who have gone before us and giving hope to those still to come. We are all connected.

Our stories make our world what it is.

Here's mine.

Still standing,

Jess Quinn

Prologue

I want you to know you are stronger than anything that tries to break you in this life. You are stronger than the battles you come up against. You are stronger than you know.

I just thought someone out there might need to hear that today.

You've got this.

IT'S THE END OF 2019, and I'm living the dream. Or I should be.

I've just stepped off a plane in Los Angeles, and I'm making my way slowly through the airport. The first time I landed here was almost ten years ago, and I was sixteen. I was expecting the coolest of cool — but, as soon as I got into the airport, I wondered if I'd somehow ended up in the wrong city. If you've ever landed at LAX, you'll know exactly what I'm talking about. The airport is dated and tired. It's dark, underground and mysterious. Everything's a mess, completely disorganised, and always apparently 'under construction'. It's like upgrades are perpetually on the way, but in all my visits I've never actually seen anything done about them. The moment you step off the plane, in desperate need of a shower, you're pulled into a below-ground world where you lose all sense of time and daylight. There's something really intimidating about it all. I always find myself feeling like I've done something wrong. The security guards almost outnumber the arriving passengers, and I feel like I have to be on my best behaviour. All I seem to be able to say is, 'Yes, ma'am. No, sir.' You spend hours waiting in lines that wind all the way to nowhere. It's enough to make you ask yourself if the twelve-hour flight back to New Zealand might be an easier option.

By now though, I've been here often enough to know that the sunshine and effortless cool of the City of Angels await me on the other side. All I have to do is get through the airport. And, when I finally step outside, I'm cocooned in a wave of SoCal warmth. It's autumn — or fall, I should say, since I'm about to officially make this my second home — but the temperature's barely any different from that of Auckland in early spring. The only difference is there's no humidity. Sweet relief.

About a year ago, I got signed to a modelling agency in LA, and it's taken me that long to sort out the paperwork I need to live and work in the States. In the meantime, I've been over quite a lot, and every time I leave knowing that I'll relocate to LA soon. Ever since my first visit, I've felt the strongest pull towards this city. I dream of living here. Who wouldn't? It's fun, it's exciting and it's full of opportunities and challenges. Here, I've finally got the chance to go hard at all the things I've spent so many years working towards. And, as I stand in front of the airport waiting for my driver (yes, I went full celebrity and ordered myself a driver — when in LA, right?), I just want to feel excited. I so badly want to be here, and I wish that all I had to think about was the adventure ahead. But right now I mostly feel like crying.

The truth is, I've never been so disheartened in my life. All my biggest dreams are waiting for me, just beyond my fingertips, but they've never felt further from my reach. Try as I might, I just can't stretch that last little distance to grasp hold of them. It's not my mind or my willpower stopping me — believe me when I say I would do anything to bridge that gap. If I could find a way to pull my dreams to me using just the power of my mind, I would. The thing that's holding me back is something I can't change. It's also the thing that, in a roundabout way, got me here in the first place: my body.

The past couple of years have been some of the most challenging I've ever lived through — and, if you know me at all, that's saying something. Don't get me wrong. I've had some of my most incredible days in that time too. It's just that the bad days have been *so* rough. I've had days when I haven't been able to get out of bed, when I can't do my job or any of the stuff I've got so used to doing, when I can't do all the things I want to do, and it's beyond infuriating. I've been living in a body that no longer feels like my own.

I so badly want to be back in the body I had just a few years ago. I don't even long for the one I had when I was a child any more. I just want the one that danced for hours on end, carried me through intense gym sessions and opened up a world of possibilities nine-year-old Jess never could have imagined.

I want to be able to live the dream I once wasn't even brave enough to have . . .

But right at this moment, when that dream is so close I can practically smell it, it's never felt so far away.

1

Puzzle pieces

They say time heals all wounds, but not every wound is the kind that heals. Some wounds grow with you. They still hurt, they stay raw, and sometimes remembering them makes them hurt in a whole new way.

My memories don't always feel like my own. Recalling some of the painful ones can feel a bit like watching it all happen to someone else. Parts don't make sense. Bits are missing. I'm overcome by this feeling I can't quite pinpoint that sits deep in the pit of my heart.

And, sure, in some ways life was cruel to me just as it was beginning, but it was also incredibly kind to me. It gave me a second chance.

So, no matter where I go, I want to leave footprints of love and kindness.

I WILL NEVER FORGET the day I went to pick up my blade.

It was a classically balmy Auckland morning when I walked into the little green-roofed building just off Dominion Road that houses the Limb Centre. By this time, the place was so familiar it felt like going to visit an old friend. I was 23, and well and truly past my teenage years, a time when I'd been so uncomfortable with my body and the ways it differs from other bodies. Today, I was proudly wearing shorts, doing nothing to hide my prosthetic leg — but not really doing anything to show it off either. Since it was designed to look as much like my other leg as possible, people often didn't notice it. I could go months after meeting someone before they even realised I had a prosthetic leg, and that was fine with me. I was confident in myself and my body, but I was also happy to be able to get through the day without being asked about it, without having to look down and get an instant reminder of all the ways I am different. This was just my way of trying not to let my leg be one of the main parts of my life and, for the past few years, it was an approach that had worked for me.

The blade was about to shake all of that up.

The idea to order myself a running blade — you know, the kind Paralympians wear — was one I'd been toying with for a while. I really, really wanted to run, but my existing prosthetic just wasn't up to the task. So I'd decided it was time to give the blade a go. Blades are specifically designed to offer a type of spring in the foot that everyday prosthetics don't, but I knew it still might not work. Even with a blade, running might remain impossible for me because, unlike most amputees I'd seen using them, I have a foot for a knee and a calf muscle for a quad. That (unsurprisingly) limits my range of motion. But I figured I could only give it a go.

As always with getting a new prosthetic, it had been quite the process. First, I'd had to get funding approved for a new leg, and then the Limb Centre had ordered the parts. These took a few months to turn up, and then everything had to be put together and custom-fitted to me. Finally, today, the blade was ready for me to try on for the first time.

As I stepped through the door, I felt a flicker of excitement. I couldn't wait to see the blade. I was beyond active at this point in my life, and I hoped it might be the tool that would help me take that further. When I first set eyes on it, I felt like I'd opened a box of fresh sneakers. I'd had it designed to look as cool as possible, and it was *very* cool. The bottom half was part-designed by Nike and had a removable sole similar to that of a running shoe. This was fitted on to the black carbon-fibre spring, then there was a black carbon-fibre socket — made just for me — with a black leather corset inside to hold my foot in place.

I put it on straight away. I looked down and felt so happy. It looked nothing at all like a leg, but it felt so much like me.

Without having even taken a step on it, I felt like an athlete.

I felt capable.

I felt super-abled.

WHENEVER PEOPLE DO NOTICE my prosthetic leg, it definitely sparks a variety of responses. Most are fascinated to hear what happened. It's a long story, and to tell it I have to go right back to the beginning.

Let's start on Sunday, 18 March 2001. A day I remember so clearly, for reasons that are about to become obvious. It was beautiful and sunny, and still warm even though the summer evenings had started to shorten. I was eight, and I was mucking around in the little playhouse in our Albany backyard with my big sister, Abby, who was ten.

Our cousins had been round for a sleepover, so it had been a busy weekend and our little sister, Sophie-Rose, who was four, was having a nap.

We loved that backyard. It seemed like an enormous playground to us, even though it was actually pretty small. I find lots of memories from childhood are like that — they're at a totally different scale from how you see things as an adult. It's like your favourite things from childhood shrink as you get bigger, but of course the only thing changing is you. When you're a kid, that tree you love climbing so much seems like the whole world. But then you grow up, and you realise the tree wasn't actually very big at all. It's just that you were really small — so small you couldn't possibly have imagined how big the world actually is.

Lots of memories from childhood are like that — they're at a totally different scale from how you see things as an adult. It's like your favourite things from childhood shrink as you get bigger, but of course the only thing changing is you.

Anyway, when we were done in the playhouse, Abby and I went out on the lawn. We mucked around with the swingball for a while, and at some point I ran off to grab a soccer ball.

'Hey, Abby!' I shouted. 'Watch this!'

Abby has always been very much the big sister in our family — equal parts relaxed around me and Soph and protective of us. Since day one, I've looked up to her and lived in her shadow, but always in the very best way possible. Once I was sure that she was watching, I put first one foot on top of the soccer ball and then the other. I was trying to stand on top of it and balance there — I'd seen other kids do it before, and had mastered it myself. Not an overly extreme activity, but I thought I was pretty talented.

'Cool!' Abby said, once I was balancing on the top.

I grinned.

Then, all of a sudden, my right leg buckled under me and I fell to the ground.

And then I screamed.

THERE ARE MOMENTS IN your life when it feels like time becomes irrelevant. It's like the whole Earth is thrown off its axis, and all the things you took for granted get shaken up and shuffled and replaced in the wrong order. Things don't make sense. You can't work out why stuff is happening the way it is. Your brain can't keep up with this altered reality, but time doesn't pause. You don't have a chance to catch up. So you hang there, frozen in a moment you couldn't possibly have seen coming, and meanwhile everything continues to move all around you. It's like you've slowed down but time has sped up, and you're stuck in between two mismatched versions of your own life.

When I look back on the moment I fell off that ball and lay there screaming on the grass, that's how it all feels. The things I remember happening immediately afterwards are like short, separate scenes, one following the other. They go something like this:

Dad appearing and scooping me up in his arms.

Mum calling the ambulance.

Abby hovering silently and watching it all, but still close enough to make sure I was okay.

My previously skinny right leg swelling in front of my eyes so much that my favourite and once-baggy early-2000s zip-side trackpants suctioned tightly around it.

Dad sitting on the couch with me on his lap, while I hugged my leg to my chest, trying not to move. Any movement — even the tiniest thing — was excruciating.

The ambulance arriving, finally.

The paramedics lying me down on a stretcher and dosing me up with laughing gas.

The paramedics cutting off my favourite trackpants so they could get to my leg.

The paramedics snapping my leg back into place so I could straighten it out again. The sound it made still sends a shudder down my spine. Thankfully, I've forgotten how it felt.

Being loaded into the ambulance with Dad, while Mum gathered Abby and Soph — who was now wide awake, thanks to all the commotion — and put them in the car to follow us.

And then the laughing gas took over.

Everything became hazy, floaty, unclear.

SOMETIMES IT FEELS LIKE my life has been one big puzzle, and writing this book has been the story of trying to put it all together. The border was easy — I already knew where the framing bits were, so all I had to do was put them in the right place. It was when I started trying to fill in the middle that I discovered some pieces were missing or didn't quite fit. Some pieces seemed like they belonged to another puzzle altogether. The thing is, I've been chipping away at this puzzle for two decades and I'm only just starting to see my story more clearly.

A huge chunk of the puzzle came together when I recently read my childhood medical records. I'd been meaning to request them for years, but it was the process of writing this book that gave me the drive to actually do it. They arrived on my doorstep in a courier package, and it was one of the heaviest parcels I've ever received. Inside were piles and piles of paper, along with CDs. As I looked at it all sitting in front of me, I got an instant flashback to attending appointments at the hospital as a kid. I'd arrive at the outpatient clinic with Mum or Dad at my side, and the nurse at reception would ask for my name and hospital number so they could get my notes out. I'd say my name and, with a laugh, point straight to the largest folder in the pile on the nurse's desk. Most kids were there for a broken-bone check-up, so their folders held only five or so pages. Mine was bigger than this book. It was comically easy to pick it out of any pile. I always thought that was funny.

As an adult, actually sitting down and reading through all those notes was a massive job. It was almost like reading someone else's story, because the truth is I have barely any recollection of a lot of what happened in the months after I fell off that ball. There were particular moments that had always stood out, but I'd never known exactly where they fitted in the puzzle. They were just floating pieces. When I started writing this book, though, I knew I had to work out where they went. I knew that, if I wanted to really understand who I am now, I had to first understand where I'd been. I wanted to know a bit more about that little girl who ended up stuck in a hospital ward. I wanted to know what she'd gone through, to learn all the things that adult me has forgotten — to put all the pieces in their rightful places. Well, I found more than I was looking for. I found answers to questions I'd never even thought to ask. I got insight not only into my own life, but also into what my parents and my sisters went through.

Whenever we remember stuff from our past, I think we tend to recall how we felt. We remember the emotions, but we don't often remember the facts. That, or somewhere along the way, as we mentally try to piece everything together, the facts slowly peel away from the truth. The feelings colour everything, and the precise details fade into the background or disappear altogether. Our life in the present moment is like a detailed line drawing, carefully coloured in, but as it moves into the past and we look back, it becomes a watercolour painting — everything blurs together.

There's no emotion in my medical notes, only facts. The cold, hard facts. And so many dates, rolling from one week into the next, and round and round in an endless loop — hospital admission, followed by discharge, followed by hospital admission, over and over again. Before I began reading my notes, I partly expected to feel overwhelmed with emotion, but I actually didn't feel anything. I just saw those facts. I guess maybe that's the way my subconscious deals with it all. I've never felt overly emotional about what I went through as a kid. I don't often look at photographs with tears rolling down my face. I don't often think of the past and cry. For a long time, I wondered whether maybe that was because my emotions were just locked away, hidden somewhere deep down beneath all the trauma. But, just like the time I sat in a therapist's chair hoping I might unlock a Pandora's box of emotions and nothing happened, my medical notes didn't crack anything open. Now, I think that the emotions I thought I was suppressing aren't actually there. Maybe it's just that those memories simply don't hurt me in the way people might expect them to. Maybe that's just how I process things, like my dad, in a matter-of-fact sort of way.

When I read my notes, I could see it all in my mind's eye. I could put my child self inside the walls of the hospital. I could see all the surgery rooms and doctors and wards. My memory of all those places and people is so clear — it's just that the events don't *feel* like they are part of my life.

It's like it all happened to someone else.

THE FIRST NOTE IN my medical records is dated the day after I fell off that soccer ball. It tells what the doctors discovered when I arrived at the hospital that Sunday afternoon, and what they did about it:

19 March 2001
Diagnosis: Fractured junction of middle and distal thirds right femur.
Operation: Intramedullary flexible nailing of right femur. The patient placed on the operating table, the leg prepped and draped.

To put that in plain English, I had broken my femur, the strongest bone in my body, also known as the thigh bone. The big one that runs between the hip and the knee.

I was sent straight to surgery, where I had rods inserted in my right leg to allow the break to heal. After the surgery, I was put in a plaster cast known as a hip spica. It went up above my waist, down the full length of my broken right leg, and down half of my other leg. Have you ever seen one of those fiddler crabs, with one normal-sized claw and one enormous one? I looked a bit like that: on the left, my skinny kid leg poked out of the plaster, and on the other side sat my right leg, totally encased in plaster and twice its actual size. This hip spica might sound like overkill — and I promise you it felt like it — but it was necessary to hold my hips in place while my femur healed. I spent a few weeks in hospital like that, followed by several more recovering at home, and it didn't take long before I was completely over it.

The plaster cast itched like crazy, and on top of that I had no independence. I had a wheelchair to get around in, but because it was extra wide to accommodate all that plaster, it was really difficult to manoeuvre through doorways. If I had to go to the bathroom in the middle of the night, I couldn't go by myself — Mum or Dad would have to come and get me and carry me there. And I was only eight years old. I wanted to get back to my life. While I was stuck in my hip spica, I was missing out. There were all these things happening beyond my couch that were incredibly important to me at that age — friends' birthday parties, netball trials, stuff like that. I desperately wanted to get back to it all.

Also, it hurt. Like, all the time. The doctors had warned that the first couple of weeks after the surgery would be painful, but they said it should then start to settle. The only thing was, it didn't. Almost three weeks later, I was still complaining about the pain, so Mum and Dad took me back to the hospital for a check-up. After doing an X-ray, the doctors decided to place me under a general anaesthetic so they could cut open my cast and have a closer look. They didn't find anything. 'Cast was removed and the skin was in excellent condition,' my notes from 11 April read.

A month went by. I was still in a lot of pain and discomfort, but I was beginning to get excited about having my cast removed. When that happened, I could finally get back to my life as I knew it. I couldn't wait. And, in the middle of May, that much-hated hip spica finally came off — but it was immediately obvious that getting back to my old life wasn't going to be quite as simple as I'd hoped.

> 17 May 2001
>
> Today, after the cast was removed, Jessica was quite apprehensive and unwilling to move her right knee. There was still some tenderness at the

fracture site. It was decided to mobilise her out of the cast and on crutches with weight-bearing as tolerated. She was reassured and we explained it was very important to start moving the knee. We will see her in three weeks.

When I first read this note and saw that word 'tenderness', I instantly remembered the feeling. It was one I've experienced a lot since that day. It's not the kind of pain you feel sharply, but the kind that's your body telling you to stop. It's the sort of twinge your body uses to protect you from worse pain.

I was appointed a physiotherapist, who was apparently going to help me get back on my feet. The goal was for me to get a full range of motion back into my injured leg so that I could eventually walk again without crutches. I spent a lot of time doing various exercises, but they all just left me in even more pain. I was making very little progress, and it was infuriating. I remember one physio session in particular from this time. I was walking on a treadmill, and every step was so uncomfortable. Whenever I placed my right foot on the moving belt, pain shot up my leg. It just felt wrong, and with every step I grew increasingly frustrated.

'Keep going, Jess,' the physio said. 'It's hard, but you can do it.'

Mum was there too. 'You're doing a really great job, honey,' she said, trying to encourage me. She could see I was getting fed up. I felt tears of annoyance pricking my eyes.

'It's normal for it to hurt a bit,' the physio added. 'You've been in a cast for a long time, and that means it's going to take time to learn to move again. Keep it up, Jess. Keep trying.'

But I *was* trying. I was trying my absolute hardest. I was doing everything the physio said. So why wasn't it working? Why was it hurting so much? Was I doing it wrong? Was it because I wasn't strong enough to push through?

I started crying out of sheer frustration, and the session ended.

I left feeling so dispirited. I just wanted to walk again.

THAT FEELING OF FRUSTRATION became a constant sidekick to my ongoing pain. The hip spica stayed off, I went back to school and I stuck at my physio, but I just didn't seem to be making any progress. I so badly wanted my broken leg to get better, but it felt like I wasn't getting anywhere. Every time I went back to the hospital for a routine check-up, I told the doctors I was still in pain. They noticed my movement around my knee was stiff, but after reviewing my X-rays they determined the fracture was healing well and sent me on my way. 'Carry on with the physio until you don't need your crutches' was essentially the message.

But, as the weeks went by, my dad started to get frustrated too. He could see how much pain I was in, and he knew it wasn't normal. So he called my doctor, who sent us back to the hospital — again.

> 9 July 2001
> Jessica attends clinic today. The father says she has
> a lot of problems with the pins. On examination,
> I can feel the pin under the skin and there is some
> irritation locally. Fusiform swelling at the site of the
> fracture, which I believe is callus formation.

They admitted me to hospital and took another X-ray and an MRI scan, just to be sure. And, three days later, I was sent into surgery once more — but the notes made ahead of that operation had suddenly changed tune. They began to tell a very different story from the one that had been unfurling up to that point. My doctors started speaking a new language altogether — one that made no sense to me at the time, but made a lot more sense of my pain.

> 12 July 2001
> It became apparent this week that Jess's fracture
> was behaving in an abnormal way. She was
> admitted to hospital and reviewed. Local staging
> included a repeat X-ray and MRI scan, which
> shows an area of bone erosion as well as a large
> soft-tissue mass at the level of the fracture site.

The suspicion therefore is this is a pathological
fracture with an underlying osteosarcoma.

The notes documenting the surgery itself go on to confirm
this suspicion: 'There was a white firm mass . . . indicative
of osteosarcoma,' they read.

Osteosarcoma.

Maybe it's a word you've heard before, maybe not. I can
tell you that, back then, at the age of eight, I'd certainly
never come across it. I could barely pronounce it, let alone
tell you what it meant. Now, though, it's almost as familiar
to me as my own name.

It was the answer to what had been causing me all that
pain for all those months. It was the reason I'd broken the
strongest bone in my body just by standing on it. It was the
reason I didn't seem to be getting anywhere with my physio.
And it wasn't a 'callus formation'. It wasn't a normal part of
the healing process.

It was cancer.

WHEN I LOOK BACK on that day now, it's my parents
I think of first. I picture them sitting in the waiting room
while I was in the operating theatre, and I can't begin to
imagine how they must have felt. Even if eight-year-old me
didn't understand what was really going on, they certainly

did. They knew what being in surgery for a biopsy meant. Their child, who only months before had been running around in the backyard, happy and healthy, laughing with her sisters and cousins, was being screened for cancer. What must have been going through their minds?

I also think of my sisters. They would have been at school, completely naive to the fact that their whole lives were about to change forever.

I guess I was up on the ward, recovering from the surgery, when Mum and Dad were called into a meeting room to be given the news once and for all: 'Your little girl has cancer.' It's a strange thought that, while they were hearing these words, I was sitting in a hospital bed happily sipping orange juice and eating jelly.

I've always wondered how my parents responded when they first got the official diagnosis. These days, if my sisters or I have even a mosquito bite that flares up, Mum goes into full care mode. Keeping us safe and healthy is her top priority. I'm sure that's partly a result of everything I went through as a kid, but it's also just the way she is. It wasn't until I read my medical notes that, for the first time, I got a rough idea of how the news affected her in particular.

13 July 2001
Referral to psych liaison. Active problems:
1. Mother distressed, shocked.

2. Child diagnosed yesterday with osteosarcoma.
Reason for referral: She was told yesterday that
Jessica has osteosarcoma, will probably need
leg amputated.

Among all of my medical notes, it was this one that broke my heart the most. At the same time as my parents found out I had cancer, they were also told I was likely to lose my leg. And until I read this all these years later, I'd always thought the plan had been for me to try to fight the cancer first, before anyone even talked about amputating my leg. That note set me straight.

Of course my mum was distressed. Of course she was shocked.

No parent should have to go through that. Ever.

But my parents did. And, what's worse, it was only the beginning.

2

Little fighter

'Play the hands you are dealt as if they are the hands you wanted.'

This is something I tell myself daily, something I've had to learn through experience. Sure, a situation may not be ideal, or what you had in mind, but you often can't change it. It's the hand you've been dealt.

Here's what you can do: adapt. It will take courage, and it will be hard, but I promise that you can do it. And, when you do adapt — once you stop spending your time resisting the change — you might just realise that life has planted you right where you were meant to be. Maybe not where you wanted to be, but definitely where you were meant to be. And maybe where you are isn't as bad as the picture you had painted in your head.

JUST OVER A WEEK after I was diagnosed with cancer, on 25 July 2001, I started chemotherapy. My doctors had planned a treatment schedule that stretched all the way to April the following year — they were really worried about the cancer spreading to other parts of my body, so the very first thing they wanted to do was to try to shrink it. I won't go into the details here, other than to say that, just three months on, the cancer had shrunk but so had I. A lot. I was a bag of skin and bones, and I had lost a drastic amount of weight along with a few other things — all my hair was gone, I could barely eat and I still couldn't walk.

The one thing I hadn't lost, apparently, was my smile. In every photo taken during that time, I've got a massive grin plastered across my face. It doesn't matter that I'm sitting in a hospital bed, hooked up to who knows how many machines, or that I've had my body poked and prodded and dissected. I'm still smiling. I look at those photos and I recognise that little fighter, because she's still inside me. I've always seen myself as having a natural optimism, no matter what the circumstances. For me, it's never been a matter of glass half full or glass half empty — what has always mattered is that I have water in my glass at all. Sometimes, that water is a small drop that I savour. Regardless of how tough it gets, even among the frustration I've always been grateful — grateful to be here, grateful to still have a life to fight for. I can see that in the photos from that time.

> **For me, it's never been a matter of glass half full or glass half empty — what has always mattered is that I have water in my glass at all.**

I might have been grinning, but behind those pictures lurked bad news: the cancer hadn't shrunk anywhere near as much as I had. It was smaller, sure, but it was still there. So, just as my doctors had indicated at the outset, it was time to talk about amputating my leg.

Usually, there would have been three options for someone with the type of cancer I had. Option one was a bone replacement, where my cancer-ridden femur would be replaced with one from a donor. While this option allows people to keep their entire leg and therefore return eventually to full mobility, it comes with a really high risk of infection and regular surgeries — something my parents were keen to avoid. When I finally left that hospital, Mum and Dad wanted me to have the highest chance possible of never having to go back in again. But that was beside the point, anyway. That option wasn't ever on the cards for me. You see, the nature of my initial break and subsequent treatment meant it was highly likely that the cancer had already spread from my femur up into my hip — so removing the femur wouldn't remove the cancer. Making sure I was cancer-free was the number-one priority, so no bone replacement for me.

The second option, then, was what's called a full hip disarticulation. This is when the leg is amputated right at, or just below, the hip socket. Doing this would have got rid of the cancer, but it would also have resulted in a lack of mobility — there's nothing left of the leg to fit a prosthetic to, so it would have meant I'd likely be on crutches or in a wheelchair for the rest of my life. Also not ideal since the next priority after getting me cancer-free was to give me the best chance at an active and independent life.

That left just one more option to explore. You might need to concentrate for this — and, if you have to read what I'm about to describe a few times over, then go away and google it; you're not alone. It can be difficult to get your head around at first, and looking at pictures helps. Option three was a procedure called a Van Nes rotationplasty or just rotationplasty — or, as I like to call it, 'backwards foot'. Basically, what happens is that most of the section of the leg between the knee and the hip is removed, then the lower section of the leg — the calf and foot — is rotated 180 degrees and reattached to what remains of the femur below the hip. In my case, because of where the cancer was located, that meant removing everything from the very top of my femur right down to below my knee. So, what was my knee joint would be replaced with my heel and ankle, while my foot would sit inside a prosthetic leg and act as a lever. This enables the patient to walk in a way that somewhat replicates the knee. The benefit to rotationplasty is that it grants the patient a much more active and independent life. The main downside is how it looks: you end up with a heel for a knee and a calf for a thigh. It isn't exactly what you'd call visually pleasing but, as you can see, the options were limited.

Since amputation had been on the cards for me since the get-go, my surgeon, Mike Hanlon, had actually begun investigating all three options before I'd even started chemo. The first thing he'd done, back in July, was to email an orthopaedic oncology surgeon in the United States to ask for their professional opinion. 'I wonder whether a modified rotationplasty procedure taking the tibia to the level of the femoral neck/head, obtaining union at this site and proceeding as per normal rotationplasty may be an option for her,' Mike wrote. 'I would welcome your thoughts on this interesting but difficult problem.'

The reason Mike was seeking advice from overseas is because, not surprisingly, rotationplasty isn't an especially straightforward procedure, and at that time only one had ever been performed here in New Zealand. That patient was a young girl too, but she had eventually passed away from other complications. And, for me, a rotationplasty would be even more complex than usual. This seems to be a common theme in my life. I guess you could say I always like to add an extra challenge.

Normally, the top of the thigh is salvaged so that the rotationplasty starts lower down — this retains more muscles and results in a slightly more visually pleasing outcome. But that wouldn't be possible for me. Due to the risk of the cancer lingering in my hip, a rotationplasty would have to be performed using only a very small section of the femur head. What that meant was that, visually, my calf-cum-thigh would sit directly under my butt. Mike wanted to know if it would still work.

A few weeks later, he got a reply. 'I think the safest option is obviously hip disarticulation,' the US surgeon wrote, 'but that rotationplasty would be a reasonably safe alternative, and could be accomplished saving the femoral head and neck. This would not leave much to gain fixation, but at

Jess's age healing should be rapid. I think it is at least worth a try.'

It's always amused me how doctors have the most incredible ability to talk in a way that removes all emotion from the equation. They really do have their own special language. All of a sudden, I was an 'interesting but difficult problem' and something that was 'at least worth a try'. I have so much respect for this capacity to simply see a situation that needs a resolution. I'll also forever be incredibly grateful to Mike, who I'm still close with today. He was willing to take a risk — a huge one — in order to give me the best chance at not just a good life, but a life full stop.

We weren't picking an ideal life. We were picking a card from the poor hand we'd been dealt. We didn't have a joker or an ace or a king to play.

ONCE MY MEDICAL TEAM had spelt out the options and given us every bit of information they could, all that remained for my parents and me was to choose which one to go with. No one wanted to pick any option. None was ideal. But then neither was the situation I was in. We weren't picking an ideal life. We were picking a card from the poor hand we'd been dealt. We didn't have a joker or an ace or a king to play. Instead, we simply had to play one of the cards we had and hope we were choosing the one that would give me the best chance of staying in the game.

'How did it feel to make that decision?' It's one of the most common questions I get asked. And honestly? It's not something I remember much of. My parents were open with me the whole way through, because they knew that it was my body and my rights — but, at the same time, I was only eight. The biggest decision I'd ever made was what Happy Meal toy I wanted at McDonald's. I simply wasn't equipped to make this kind of choice. So that meant it fell to Mum and Dad.

When I asked Dad about it recently, he said it was never a matter of whether or not to amputate. 'We would never have been brave enough to argue against it, as we would have hated to have made the call and then lost you,' he said. The choice was one of which approach to take: rotationplasty or disarticulation? Even then, it wasn't black and white. As Dad's since explained to me, Mike wasn't actually 100 per cent certain he could make a rotationplasty work. He told my parents he wouldn't know that until I was already in surgery and he had removed my leg. It all depended on how high the cancer had gone and whether or not there'd be enough of the top of my leg left to reattach my rotated calf to. The best Mike could propose was that he could begin to operate as though he was doing a rotationplasty, then change to a disarticulation if he discovered that wasn't going to work.

Outside of my medical team, there was no one else we could look to for advice here in New Zealand — no one who'd had a rotationplasty, no one to tell us how successful it might be, no one to help us weigh the pros and cons. This was 2001, remember. You couldn't just pop on Instagram and search #rotationplasty, then message people around the world. Yahoo did exist, though, and Dad put that to good use. Through his extensive searching, he somehow managed to find a young girl in Canada who'd been through the procedure. I remember we got a copy of a book she'd written that showed how the surgery worked, which helped a bit, but that was pretty much it.

Talk about taking a stab in the dark.

It's beyond me how you even start to try to decide what to do in a situation like that, but my parents did it. They had to. And they settled on the brave choice — or, as they would say, the only choice: to at least give a rotationplasty a shot.

I take my hat off to them every day for making that call, and I hope more than anything that I have lived a life that shows they did the right thing. I don't recall feeling upset when I learnt what the plan was. Perhaps it's just slipped from my memory, or maybe I was protected by my naivety. It could simply be that I'd become so used to the not-so-normal being normal that nothing really surprised me any more. Truly, though, I think I just had no real understanding of the reality I was facing.

If I was put in that same situation today, I don't know what I would do. I know too much now. I fear too much. I wouldn't want to disfigure my body at all. And I can't ignore the fact that the way my leg looks would be a huge factor — as a grown woman, I think I'd struggle to get past that. But to settle for a life where I couldn't do the things I want to do? Well, that would be impossible to overlook. If I had even a small chance at being able to carry on doing the things I love, I'd have to take it, no matter what. At the end of the day, your appearance really means nothing when it's a choice between how you look and your ability to move through the world at your own pace.

If I had even a small chance at being able to carry on doing the things I love, I'd have to take it, no matter what.

WHEN I WAS WHEELED into the operating ward on Thursday, 25 October 2001, I was just under a month shy of turning nine. And yet that's the day I still think of as my 'rebirthday'. It's the day that drew a line between my life 'before' and my life 'after'.

That morning in the ward, I'd given Mum and Dad a photo album I'd made with a family friend, Mary-Rose. A few weeks earlier, Mary-Rose had come and picked me up and we'd gone to the beach for a photo shoot. I'd got dressed for the occasion in head-to-toe purple (must have been my colour of the moment), and I'd had fun. That's all it was to me: a fun day out. On the way back to Mary-Rose's afterwards, we'd stopped and got the photos printed, then we stuck them in a fancy black photo album. Well, when I finally gave the album to my parents on the morning of my surgery, Mum instantly started crying. Now, as an adult, I understand why — the significance of that photo album is incredibly obvious — but I didn't get that at the time. At eight, I just didn't understand that I'd given my parents an album of what could have been, quite possibly, some of their daughter's last happy moments — or, at the very least, the last images of her body in one piece.

At some point, a nurse came in and drew on my right leg with a big black vivid. Why? To make sure the surgical team didn't take the wrong one off. (Not a mistake you want made, right?) Then she said, 'It's time for us to head down to the operating theatre now.'

That's when I said goodbye to Mum, but Dad came with me. He walked along beside my bed, holding my hand the whole way. I remember being wheeled down a long corridor, and that was when it hit me. It was like I'd suddenly, properly grasped what was about to happen, and I was scared. I was so scared. I began crying hysterically.

Dad just squeezed my hand. 'It will be okay,' he said calmly. Then he repositioned Bunny, who was tucked in beside me, so that he was closer to my heart — Bunny had been given to me on the day I was born and was with me for every surgery, blood test and chemo session.

My dad's ability to reassure me in such a scary situation will always be incredible to me. He has always had the most gentle way of handling the toughest situations. Whatever he was going through in that moment, you never would have guessed it from how he looked on the outside. (And, funnily enough, when I was recently talking about this moment with him, he said he had no recollection of me being in hysterics. Instead, he was surprised at how calm I was. So maybe we just choose to remember the things that hurt the least to relive? I know that, for me, seeing Dad's pain would have hurt more than feeling my own pain did.)

When we got to the theatre, I was transferred to the operating table. The room was full of hustle and bustle — nurses busy prepping everything, machines beeping, doctors talking — but it was also, somehow, silent. It was like it was both full of movement and deathly still at the same time. Time pooled in the same way it had when I'd very first broken my femur. I can still recall exactly how it felt. It was extremely eerie.

The anaesthetist came over to say hello, then launched into the usual small talk about my favourite TV shows — but I was all too good at this by then. I knew he was just distracting me until the anaesthetic kicked in. I knew he was being deliberately cheery to try to set me at ease, to make me feel like this was any other day. I knew it was not any other day.

Dad was still holding my hand when I felt my body begin to grow limp.

Then everything went dark.

FOURTEEN HOURS LATER, I woke up.

In that time — the shortest fourteen hours of my life, and probably the longest of my parents' — my whole body had changed. So had my world. It had all changed, irreversibly, forever.

In the end, Mike had been able to perform the rotationplasty and, given the circumstances, the surgery itself had worked out as well as could have been hoped. Even so, it would take years for my parents and my medical team to find out whether the risk they'd taken had paid off.

Just four hours after my surgery, though, we got a snippet of hope. I was in the intensive care unit, hooked up to breathing tubes and heart-rate monitors, when Mike came by to check on everything. My legs — well, the 1.5 legs I now had — were plastered up in another hip spica, with my newly backwards toes poking out the bottom of the right side. Mike touched them to check the blood circulation, and I wiggled them. I moved my toes the way anyone would move their toes, just backwards.

To this day, that blows my mind.

A whole section of my body had been dismantled and put back together in a way that no human body was ever designed to be assembled. My nerves had all been put in places they did not belong, in the hope — and, I'm sure, after incredibly careful medical planning — that they would still function. My muscles had been cut, repositioned and reconnected. And somehow my brain just made sense of it all almost immediately.

My body had already started to adapt.

ADAPTABILITY IS SOMETHING THAT has always fascinated me. The way we, as humans, can and will adapt to unforeseeable situations or environments in ways we never dreamt possible. It's powerful, this ability. But it's a power we often don't even know we have until something happens to abruptly put us in a new place — a place we can't see working, a state that makes no sense. With time, though, we do adapt. We must. And we forget that our lives were ever different.

I don't think we give ourselves enough credit for this incredible capacity to pick up and keep going when we're forced to. We all have this power inside us, and it's there whether we know it or not. But it's an ability we need to recognise and embrace. The power itself might be innate, but using it isn't. My toes might have wiggled mere hours after my surgery, but they weren't the only part of me that needed to adapt. *All* of me needed to adapt. Everything had changed, and that meant I needed to change too.

Too often, we're so afraid of the 'bad' things change might bring into our lives that we fail to see that change also holds the potential for greatness. It's only by riding through the discomfort, by letting the change happen, that you can see it might contain some good.

We had always known this surgery would alter my life dramatically. That had been one of my parents' biggest fears — just how much it would change things for me. Change is uncomfortable, for all of us. We get used to the way things are, and we find safety in what we know. Then something comes along that shakes up our world, and it's so scary that we resist it. We want things to go back to how they were. Too often, we're so afraid of the 'bad' things change might bring into our lives that we fail to see that change also holds the potential for greatness. It's only by riding through the discomfort, by letting the change happen, that you can see it might contain some good. It might even promise more than anything you could have imagined before it came into your world.

Of course, it's easy for me to say this as I sit here and write this two decades later, with my backwards leg and knowing how things worked out, but it's also honest for me to say it. None of this has been easy, but the good that change has ultimately brought into my life has completely outweighed any of the hardships. While I can say that now, it still took me time to learn to adapt to situations I have no control over. At times, I have tried to fight the change. I have tried to fit my new life into the mould of my old life. To put it bluntly, for a while I spent a lot of time and effort trying to be a girl with two legs, when the reality was that I was a girl with one.

Before getting cancer and losing my leg, I had been a really athletic kid. I mean, even the transition from my old life to this completely new one happened the moment I stood on a soccer ball. I was always in the top netball team, I danced, I played every sport possible and I ran. It was running that was really my thing. I won all my school cross-country races, sprinting over the finish line miles ahead of anyone else, and before I got sick I'd started racing competitively outside of school. I just loved everything about running — I was a kid, and it was fun, and I was good at it. It was as simple as that. Sure, I was only eight so it's hard to say I was an athlete, but I truly couldn't get enough of anything outdoors or to do with sports. I could never have imagined myself not being able to do all the things I loved most, until one day I physically couldn't.

I was so excited the day I got fitted with my first prosthetic leg. I was the first person in New Zealand to have a prosthetic built for a rotationplasty, but as a little kid I didn't really understand what that meant. It's only with time that the consequences of being such a medical rarity have become all too real to me. About two or three years after having my surgery, I began mentoring other kids who might also have a rotationplasty done. I'd go along to show them what my leg looked like, and I think there are something like ten of us in New Zealand now — it's still not exactly commonplace. But at the age of nine, I was totally unaware of the ramifications of all of that. I just couldn't wait to get my shiny new leg on. I thought it would instantly give me back all the things I had been missing ever since my femur broke — the netball, the running, the birthday parties, the playground antics, the playing on the beach with my sisters. The me I knew before.

There are photos of me sitting in the Limb Centre, grinning from ear to ear while the prosthetist tells me all about my new leg. I hung on his every word. The leg was small, like I was, with a socket to house my foot and a long leather brace that would hug my new 'thigh' (as in, my calf muscle). The prosthetist showed me how you did it up with a thick shoelace-like cord that pulled the leather together into something resembling a corset. It looked like an artefact from the 1800s. It would have been right at home in a museum.

Yes! I have a new leg! I vividly remember thinking. *Let's get back to my life!*

In my mind, a leg was a leg. How hard could it be? You just put it on and then you walked, right?

It wasn't anywhere near as simple as that. A leg made out of carbon fibre and plastic reacts very differently from one of flesh and bone. First, I had to learn how to put the leg on, then I had to learn how to use it. That meant relearning everything I had once known how to do so well, but this time I had to do it in a body that no longer felt familiar to me in any way. No one — least of all that grinning kid sitting in the Limb Centre — could have imagined just how enormous this task would be.

I took my shiny new leg home, and my new routine began. Each morning, Mum or Dad would come into my room and help me put my leg on. They'd lace each bit up, then gently help me stand and get myself braced against my crutches. Every evening, we'd do the same in reverse. Luckily, it didn't take me long to get confident enough on my crutches that I could return to school. Sure, I looked like a baby giraffe about to topple at any minute, crutches and legs going in every direction at once, but I didn't care.

I was just so happy to be back with my friends. My shiny new leg was a novelty, and even if every fall — and there were many — caused excruciating pain because my wound and my nerves were still so raw, I was determined to get around on it. Over the year, I gradually ditched first one crutch, then both, until I was able to walk on my own two feet (well, three if you want to get technical about it). There were still lots of things I couldn't do — play the sports I used to, run around with my friends, participate in egg-and-spoon races at birthday parties — but I never worried too much about any of that. Anything was better than being in hospital.

It's early days, I thought. *I'll be able to do those things again soon.*

I've always been grateful for the naivety I had as a child. It allowed me to just get on with it without even thinking about the implications this would all have for my future.

I didn't dwell on what I couldn't do. I just got on with it. And that meant, to begin with, I bounced back really quickly. Neither my parents nor my doctors had been sure what to expect. They'd had no idea how I would transition back to life. Looking back, we had nothing to worry about. I've always been grateful for the naivety I had as a child.

It allowed me to just get on with it without even thinking about the implications this would all have for my future.

Mobility had been one of the deciding factors in trying for a rotationplasty, and it definitely gave me abilities that I might never have had otherwise, but that doesn't mean it was easy. Or ideal. At the age of nine, I'd had my body rearranged in a way that still makes even the most seasoned professionals stare a little blankly and scratch their heads. Even now, I'll sometimes get out of the bath, dry myself off, and sit and stare and think, *I have the most unusual body.* There was no guidebook called 'How to Do Life with a Backwards Foot for a Knee'. There was no one to look to for reference. I *was* the reference. For each new experience or challenge I faced, I was the guinea pig. That's still true to this day.

From the moment I got moving on my new leg, I was determined to find something that would give me the same sense of satisfaction I'd once got from sports. I tried absolutely everything I could think of. I gave learning to play the guitar a go. I took golf lessons — it was, I figured, still a sport, just one that offered a less intense approach. I even tried competitive table tennis. But nothing stuck. Nothing came close to giving me what running, dancing and team sports once had.

One sunny weekend when I was about eleven, Dad saw how frustrated I was and decided he'd try to help. I've never known how he works it out, but he always does. 'Look,' he said. 'Why don't we go up to the school and have a go at running?'

Now, my dad has never been the athletic type. Not at all. But he would do anything to help me. If I'd said, 'Dad, I want to run ten kilometres but only if you do it with me,' he would have done it.

The school was only five minutes' walk from our house, and when we reached the sports field behind the classrooms I looked out over the green grass. I used to run around on it without a second thought, but that once familiar space now seemed dauntingly big. I started walking around the outside, then I slowly picked up the pace. Then I tried to run, but the best I could manage was a sort of skip-hop manoeuvre. Dad was by my side the whole way, doing his best to explain things step by step. But how do you even begin to explain something that you do on autopilot? Trying to talk someone else through an action you do largely by instinct is nearly impossible. It all stops making sense. It's like telling someone to 'act natural' when you're taking a photo of them, and suddenly they don't know what to do with their arms or their hands and instead they do something incredibly awkward.

It's even harder trying to explain how to do something that your instinct thinks your body is capable of when your body has changed. It's like trying to drive a car whose battery has been disconnected. You know how to make it work in theory, but it just won't do what you're asking it to do. That's what running was like for me. I'd spent almost nine years of my life with two legs and I'd known how to run on them, but suddenly my body couldn't do that any more. In my mind's eye, it seemed so easy — I felt like I knew exactly what I needed to do and I could see myself running — but when I tried to make my body match what I felt inside, it just wouldn't work. It all fell apart.

I gave it everything that day on the field, but I couldn't get past that skip-hop. As we left, I was quiet. Dad knew I was frustrated.

'We'll come back next weekend,' he said. 'We'll keep working on it.'

And we did. But every weekend the same thing happened. It wasn't lack of coordination that was the problem, but my prosthetic. It was impossible to try to do anything quickly with a foot that simply wasn't made to move like my good leg did.[1] The prosthetic lacked all the stuff that gives you the ability to run — there was no natural ankle flexion, no ability to spring up, and no connection to knee, quad and glute. Before long, my frustration gave way to deflation. It

---

1 For ease, and since that's what I called it when I was a kid, you might notice that I sometimes refer to my left leg as my 'good' leg — but that's not to say I think my right leg isn't good. At the end of the day, they're both good legs, but I also need an easy way to distinguish between them, and this is just the way that's always worked for me.

was disheartening to keep trying so hard and not gain any ground, so I gave up.

'I can't run,' I told myself.

AS I GOT OLDER, I started to get a clearer perspective on just how many challenges I might face living in this differently abled body. Things started to get harder, and that was my first clue to just how turbulent life can be. It's never either easy or hard. Usually, it's a combination of both, but it took growing up for me to realise that. I think this is probably true for a lot of us. We mature, we develop fears and the golden paint on our childhood world begins to chip.

As one year passed, then another and another, what had at first been shiny and new just became normal. It was no longer enough that I'd survived cancer or that I was out of the hospital. The shine of my leg well and truly dulled.

We mature, we develop fears and the golden paint on our childhood world begins to chip.

That leg hurt. It left blisters and rubbed my skin so raw it bled inside my prosthetic. It caused nerve pain so bad I had to be medicated. It had to be laboriously attached to my body each morning and removed each night. I became increasingly aware that it simply wasn't made for so many of the things I'd once loved. I began to properly understand the full implications of just how my life had changed — much more than I had when it had actually happened.

By the time I was at high school and into my teens, I'd stopped the rehab I'd so diligently attended for the first few years after losing my leg. I just reached a point where I wanted to put my leg and everything I had been through as far behind me as I could. I didn't want to receive daily treatment. I didn't want to always be stuck in a rehab space. I just wanted to live my life. Specifically, I started to want my old life back.

Don't get me wrong — I have always had so much love for my life, whatever shape it takes. I've fought too hard for it to let it go. It's just that, for a period of time during my teenage years, I didn't want to live like this, in this body. I remember sitting on the sidelines during PE classes, watching my peers moaning and groaning their way through beep tests and wishing so badly I could be in their place. The frustration of not being able to participate became so much that I stopped doing PE altogether, just so I didn't have to watch others doing the things I wanted to do.

It was during this time that I decided to give netball another go. I knew I could no longer fill the midcourt position I'd played before losing my leg, as that involved a lot of running, so I spent hours practising my shooting. I got to the point where I could shoot a ball through the hoop from anywhere within the goal circle. I might not have been able to move very well on the court, but damn, I could shoot. And getting that ball through the hoop was, after all, the aim of the game. I never thought I'd get into a top team again, but given my shooting prowess, I thought I at least had a chance at making a decently ranked one.

The stark reminder of where I had once been and where I now found myself stung. Every time I saw my name at the bottom of the list, I just wanted my old life back.

Every year, though, the team list would come out, and every year I'd find my name right at the bottom, assigned to Team Ten. I persevered through weekly practices and games with teammates who could barely catch the ball, and I'd head home every evening after school and practise shooting until it got so dark I couldn't see the hoop any more. I was convinced that if I could just shoot a little better, I would soon find my name higher up on the team list. If I practised hard enough, I could get my name where it used to be. But year after year it stayed right at the bottom. The stark reminder of where I had once been and where I now found myself stung. Every time I saw my name at the bottom of the list, I just wanted my old life back. I was doing everything I could and it still wasn't enough, because I was living in a body that wouldn't move in the way I wanted it to. The frustration got to me, and I gave up on netball.

But if there's one thing I am, it's stubborn. There's no telling me I can't or shouldn't do something. That will only make me more determined to do it. This might be part of why I struggled so much during my teens, but I also know it's what got me through in the end. It's what made me embrace the change. I was determined to find a way to move, no matter what, and I refused to get in my own way. That was how I finally realised that the more I tried to step into my old shoes, the harder life was going to be. It was like repeatedly trying to force a big round peg into a very small square hole. No matter how many different ways I tried to make that peg fit, it just wouldn't go in.

So I let go. I stopped trying to get my old life back, and instead I decided to focus on the life I had. There's this one story my dad loves to tell that kind of perfectly illustrates this. We were in the kitchen together, and I was telling him all about how frustrated I was because I couldn't do something (neither of us can actually remember exactly what it was — probably riding a bike or similar). I was clearly upset. But then Dad says it's like I suddenly snapped myself out of it.

'I've just got to get over myself and get on with it,' I said.

'Jess, it's okay to be frustrated,' he told me. 'You're allowed to feel pissed off.'

But he says it was clear I'd made my mind up. I'd turned my stubbornness to my own advantage, and that was that. I put my frustration to bed, and decided to concentrate on living my life. Dad has honestly told me this story so many times. He says it was my drive to just move on that really stuck with him. It was obvious that something big changed for me that day.

So I let go. I stopped trying to get my old life back, and instead I decided to focus on the life I had.

As soon as I decided to get on with it, everything started to make sense. I couldn't change anything about what had happened. I couldn't rewrite the story to have it turn out differently, with me in a different body and living a different life. At the end of the day, this is my body. As unusual as it is, as disfigured and painful and frustrating as it is, it's mine. Without this body, I wouldn't still be standing. I wouldn't be living this life.

How can I argue with that?

And you know what else? I *wouldn't* change a thing, even if I could. This is who I am. The adversity I've faced might objectively suck, but it's part of my story. We don't get to avoid adversity. That's just not realistic — adversity comes for all of us, in some shape, at some point.

What we *do* get is a choice. We can choose how we respond to what life throws at us.

That's not to say letting go is easy — but no one ever told me things were going to be easy. You have to be brave if you're going to adapt. You will probably feel yourself resisting the change, like I did, but in my experience that's your biggest clue that it's time. If you're up against a wall and you're forced to pick from a bum hand of cards you don't want to play, you still have to choose something. That's the moment you need to stop fighting, stop resisting. Yes, it's scary. It's daunting. It's full of what ifs. But how will you know what's possible if you pass instead of playing?

Choose something.

3

No hiding

Lots of people get to choose when, and if, they'll share their scars with others. They can wait to build trust and a connection with another person before they put everything on show. That's never really been an option for me, because I wear my biggest scars on the outside.

This has been both a blessing and a curse. Lots of us want to hide from our insecurities. We'd rather suppress them until we're almost numb, but our insecurities don't go away — they just wait to confront us later in life when it all gets too much.

I want to tell you something: your insecurities are nothing but roadblocks. When you reach the end of your life, you won't regret all the things you went ahead and did in spite of what others might have thought about you. What you will regret are all the moments you missed out on because you were busy hiding.

I'm not perfect. I'm still learning this one. As I overcome one insecurity, I inevitably find myself hiding behind another. These are walls I'm forced to repeatedly break down. The confidence isn't always there, but I'm still going to show up exactly as I am, no hiding away.

TOWARDS THE END OF high school, a friend who was working in a gym offered me a membership trial. Within two weeks, I was hooked. Finally, I had found an environment where I could work to my own abilities, where I could compete with myself, where I got the same sense of satisfaction that sport had once given me, where it didn't matter whether I could run or not.

I got myself a personal trainer, and each week I worked on building my strength. I also started doing rehab again — but I incorporated it into my gym work and made it what I wanted it to be. The few years of rehab I'd done had been filled with strength and functional training, but I'd always had to do it at physio clinics and hospitals — places where I felt like a patient. In the gym, I felt like everyone else. I didn't feel 'less than' or incapable.

Before I knew it, I was strong. I was moving and training like an athlete. I was boxing, lifting weights and doing intense circuit training. The gym became a place for me that wasn't about what my body looked like, but about what my body could do. Here, I was able to push myself and find new ways of doing things. Every week I got better, stronger. Within a couple of years, I could do almost anything at the gym.

When I left high school and started at uni, I began having physio again. I'd been getting migraines and neck pain, and someone recommended a place called Flexa Clinic, a privately owned physio and fitness studio. As soon as I visited, I knew it was an environment I wanted to be in. There was a gym, treatment rooms and a team of specialists who could offer me rehab disguised in a form that didn't feel like hospital. The other gym-goers were athletes and everyday people who were also going through their own rehab. I signed up and started working with physio and owner Murray Hing. For a year or so, we just worked on addressing my neck and head pain, but once that improved I began to incorporate my work at Flexa with my gym training.

I began to feel the need to push myself further, but I kept hitting up against my inability to run. Whenever I wanted to push myself, it was the one thing that would hold me back. I still dreamt of being able to run. I would drive past people out for a run and slow down a bit (probably quite creepy, in hindsight) just so I could get a closer look at the angle of their legs. Sometimes I would just sit and watch people running and think about how freeing that must feel. Whenever I was out shopping and a kid would run past me, bursting with happiness and joy, I couldn't help but feel a flash of envy. I was envious of their ability to just pick up the pace like that, and I also envied their totally carefree attitude.

When I mentioned my desire to run again, people would sometimes try to comfort me by saying, 'Oh, trust me. You're not missing out on anything!' And sure, running isn't for everyone. But that's the thing: running *was* for me. I had loved it. And I was sure I would still love it if only I could find a way to do it. Maybe if my life had taken a different path, my love of running might have eventually faded. Who knows? But I never actually got the chance to find out — that ability got taken away from me before I could know that, and that left me stuck in a kind of limbo where one of the things I remembered enjoying so much in my old body was no longer a thing I could do. I'm not suggesting everyone who has both their legs should go for daily runs in order to appreciate them, but I do know what a gift it is to be able to do something simply because you want to.

So, I went to Murray and I told him I wanted to give running another go. 'I've been thinking about getting a running blade,' I explained, 'but I know I'm going to need help to get moving on it. Can you help?'

Murray agreed.

And that's when I went ahead and ordered the blade.

THE FIRST DAY I took my blade to Flexa Clinic was pretty confronting. I had been waiting such a long time for it to be built that I was impatient to get it out on the gym floor and start putting it through its paces, but I was also nervous about stepping out in public with a leg that no longer looked anything like a leg. Wearing it inside the Limb Centre had been fine, but putting it on in the gym was a whole other matter. It almost felt like I was having to go out naked.

I walked in past the reception desk, carrying my blade in one hand and my gym bag in the other.

I headed straight to the changing room, where I set everything down on a bench.

I undressed.

Sat down and removed my old prosthetic.

Put it in the locker.

Grabbed the blade from the bench beside me.

Put the blade on.

Put my shorts and singlet on.

Tied my hair back.

Pulled my gym shoe out of my bag, then put it on my left foot.

Bent over and laced up my shoe.

Sat up.

Took a deep breath.

Stood up.

Walked out of the changing room.

Stepped onto the gym floor.

I felt off balance. I mean, I had one leg and one spring. My running blade is deliberately longer than my left leg, as it needs to have space to compress and then spring me back up when I run. This means that standing or walking with it is always really uncomfortable because my hip is hitched higher on one side. So it felt unusual, sure, but the naked feeling I'd been worried about? It wasn't there. In fact, I felt the opposite. For the first time in nearly fifteen years, I felt more 'me' than I ever had.

I could see no questions in people's faces. There was no more *I wonder why that girl is limping . . . Is that a knee brace or . . .?* Instead, it was more *That girl has one leg . . . Cool.*

I felt the biggest weight come off my shoulders. It took changing from a leg that looked like a leg to one that was a marvel of carbon fibre, but in that moment a bubble popped — one that I'd been living in without even knowing it. It took putting on my blade to make me even realise that I'd been hiding anything with my old prosthetic. That's when I understood that, sometimes, we hide our insecurities without even knowing we're doing it. Hiding becomes something so subconscious that it's hidden even to ourselves. It just takes a massive jolt or a forced confrontation with ourselves for us to realise what it is we are hiding from.

EARLIER, I SAID THAT seeing my blade for the first time was like opening a fresh box of sneakers, and that comparison's fitting in more ways than one. Prosthetics are like shoes in the sense that you need to break them in before they become comfortable and familiar. The only difference? Prosthetics require a lot more time.

> At first, I hate the leg and I'm convinced I've done the wrong thing. Then, after weeks, it starts to become a bit more familiar and I begin to forget what my old leg felt like.

It's not just a matter of getting the fit right. Once that new leg is strapped on, you have to start building the muscles you'll need to move with it. You need to allow time for your nerves to flare up and readjust. Then there are the inevitable blisters you'll get before the calluses all re-form in the right places. I go through the same process every time I get a new leg, or even if there's a minor adjustment made to a current one. At first, I hate the leg and I'm convinced I've done the wrong thing. Then, after weeks, it starts to become a bit more familiar and I begin to forget what my old leg felt like. Finally, after going through all the minute and painful physical adjustments that occur over days and months, I'll try on my old leg one day and realise just how comfortable the new one has become. I've been through this routine so many times in my life that it's basically second nature. Given all the life practice I've had in rehab, I often joke that I could probably skip the first few years of a physio degree.

I've also reached a stage, more than two decades on from having cancer and losing my leg, where I know my body inside and out. This level of self-awareness can be infuriating at times — sometimes I just want to turn it off, to not think so much about what I'm feeling physically — but at the same time I don't know how I would have made it through all the challenges life has thrown me without the unnervingly close relationship I have with my own body.

Adjusting to the blade was a little different from any other prosthetic I'd had, though. The blade was never made to be a permanent leg — it was specially designed to be used for a very specific activity. That meant I'd have to use it alongside my daily prosthetic, changing into the blade whenever I needed it. Sometimes, I might have to change legs several times a day, and that naturally made it harder to adjust to. So, during the months it had taken for my blade to be built, Murray and I had put together an intensive training plan to get me where I wanted to be in order to run. Before we even began, Murray made things really clear to me.

'Jess,' he said, knowing I'd be eager to run straight away, 'it's going to be a slow process. It's going to take time.'

Specifically, it was going to take nine months.

We had a lot of work to do — and it all started that day I first wore the blade onto the gym floor. It was literally a case of learning to walk before you run.

First, I would need to get used to the sensation of the blade and the way my foot sat in the new socket. Then, I would start to practise putting weight on it. This part was going to take a while, as my foot needed time to form new calluses and my hypersensitive nerves had to adjust to the new prosthetic. Next, I would need to strengthen all the muscles I hadn't used for fifteen years. I'd also have to work on completely rewiring how I put my weight on my leg.

We had a lot of work to do — and it all started that day I first wore the blade onto the gym floor. It was literally a case of learning to walk before you run. I spent every day in that studio. Often, I'd do two sessions a day — one at the gym before work and one at Flexa after — including both physical training and recovery physio. It was tedious stuff, but it was the kind of challenge I enjoyed. I had a purpose.

I was moving my body, training like an athlete, and I couldn't have been happier.

I specifically remember working on balancing on the blade. This was important to help my body adjust to the load it would need to bear on that side when I started running. I'd stand in front of a mirror, slowly shifting my weight onto my blade and then lifting my good leg off the floor. The goal? To balance on the blade alone for 30 seconds. That might not sound like a lot, but to begin with I couldn't even lift my left leg off the ground. It was a slow build. Each week, I would add one more second, then one more. Slowly but surely, my balance grew.

As I got stronger and realised I was getting somewhere, I started to have fun with it. One day I arrived at training a little early so that, when Murray came to meet me on the gym floor, I was already there, balancing on my leg like I'd been doing it my whole life. I kept it up for way longer than 30 seconds. I was completely showing off, just because I could.

After I nailed the balancing bit, I started moving. First up was a running-style motion that Murray demonstrated first, and then it was my turn. Trying to mimic him took me right back to being on the school field with Dad. It looked so easy when Murray did it, but every time I tried to shift my own weight in the same way, my coordination wouldn't quite match it. But I kept at it, and eventually I got there.

I was basically imitating running, but without the speed or the load.

I did this and my other strengthening exercises for months. For the most part, I loved this process of learning how to do something from scratch. It's always been the hard work that goes in during the months and years before an athlete actually competes in the main event that I've most admired. The main event is just the cherry on top. I guess I relate because I've had to spend so many years getting my body to a place where it can move in the way I want it to. I know how much time and dedication goes into reaching an ambitious physical goal. An athlete can't just turn up to an event and expect to do well without having already put in the hard work. It was the same for me after I lost my leg: I couldn't just expect to start walking, let alone running, the next day. I had to do the hard work first.

It's always been the hard work that goes in during the months and years before an athlete actually competes in the main event that I've most admired. The main event is just the cherry on top.

But, while I was loving training this way, I was also eager to just finally run. Almost every day, I asked Murray, 'So, can I have a go at running now?' His answer was always the same: 'Not yet.' I knew I had to be patient and keep training, but that wasn't always easy because I was having to put all these hours into mastering a task that so many other people never even have to think about. Where others I knew could just pick up and run, I was having to relearn how to do it excruciatingly slowly. People often ask me, 'What's the hardest thing about your leg and what you've been through?' and it's this: living in a body that doesn't always accurately connect to my mind. It felt like going back to square one, and that's because I essentially had. I was having to relearn something I'd once known, but this time I had to teach myself to do it in a completely new way. It's like I was a ballerina on pointe shoes who suddenly started training to be a runner, but with a mind that knew how to run only by balancing on her toes. Sound confusing? It was.

This is, I've learnt, the nature of having one half of a body part somewhere it wasn't made to be and the other half fabricated out of plastic and carbon fibre. Many bodies adjust to change really easily. They move and they grow, but a quarter of mine — my prosthetic — doesn't. It's also the nature of having a personality that likes to push the limits. I'm just not one to shy away from a challenge. I was never handed an easy path, so why wish for one? And, thanks to my gym training, I knew the only way to get to where I wanted to be was to compete solely with myself. It just wasn't worth making the comparison between what I could do and the abilities of others. No one else I knew had a heel for a knee. No one else I knew had ever had to teach their toes to take the whole weight of their body backwards. Comparing myself with others would be a waste of time.

I had a choice: level up, or give up.

NINE MONTHS AFTER I got my blade, in January 2016, Murray finally agreed to let me try to run.

Those tedious months of training had paid off, and I'd become really accustomed to the blade. I was comfortable moving around on it. I was ready.

While Murray watched, I walked to the other side of the gym.

Then, I put one foot in front of the other and I ran.

I ran to the opposite end of the room, and then I turned around and ran back.

I'll never forget how it felt.

I felt free.

I felt like I could do anything I wanted in this world.

All up, it was only about 50 metres across carpet and a very light jog, but none of that mattered. All that mattered was that I ran. I did something I had come to believe I would never be able to do again — something that, for so many years, had kept me sitting on the sidelines and at the bottom of team lists.

I'd done it.

But, me being me, I decided to take it even further. I wasn't going to settle for anything other than a massive challenge, so I set an even bigger goal: by the end of the year, I told myself, I was going to run ten kilometres.

Doing the things you always said you would is less of a conscious choice and more a product of the opportunities that arise as you travel whatever path you're on.

ONE OF THE INTERESTING things about writing a book is that you're constantly looking back over your own life. In hindsight, you start to see a pattern where one thing leads to the next, even though you had no idea where it was all going at the time. You understand that doing the things you always said you would is less of a conscious choice and more a product of the opportunities that arise as you travel whatever path you're on.

It makes me think of something my dad said to me when I was still in high school. 'You've just got to trust the process of life,' he said. 'Every opportunity leads to another, and you just have to follow your gut. You don't have to have it all sorted out, but one day you will look back and see that all the dots connect.'

His words that day stuck. They usually do. And he's going

to high-five himself right about now, but he was right.

Back in 2016, the year I first ran on my blade, I had just finished my uni studies — I'd got a degree in fashion and product design, and was working full-time as a product designer. I'd loved my studies and really enjoyed my job, but I'd always said that I was going to 'do something with my story' when I was older. I wasn't sure what that 'something' was, but I just had this sense that everything that I'd been through would serve a greater purpose. I'm not sure what I meant by 'older', either. It's not like you flick a switch and go from younger to older overnight. Growing up happens gradually. It's only when you're already there that you realise that maybe you're 'older' now.

Before I'd got my blade, I'd thought the whole process of learning to run was just about movement and my abilities, but the blade ended up being about so much more than that. Right from the first time I tried it on, it lifted me to a new level of confidence — one where I felt totally happy and proud to be myself. The blade showed me what I'd been hiding, and got me started down the road of sharing more openly everything that made my experience and my body unique.

One day, a talented photographer friend, Jono Parker, and I got talking about projects we could work on together. 'It'd be so fun to do a shoot with you wearing your blade,' he said.

I was really into the idea. 'Let's do it,' I said.

So we got another friend, Courtney Perham, who I studied with and who has an amazing sense of style, on board to style the shoot. We didn't really have any intentions for what would come of it — we just felt like it would be a bit of fun. In the back of my mind I thought that if the photos came out okay it might be cool to send them to a modelling agency. This wasn't because I had any aspirations of being a model. In fact, I didn't really like getting my picture taken at all. Instead, I'd started in recent years to become aware of the opportunity my body could represent. While studying fashion, I'd become increasingly puzzled by the fact that professional models represented only a very small part of the population, and that meant they always looked the same.

As a kid, I'd pretty quickly got used to never seeing anyone in advertising who looked like me — that was, I figured, just the way the cookie crumbled for me. In my mind, it didn't make sense, but I also never thought I had the power to challenge it. I figured it was just the way it was. But as I got older, I began to realise that lots of people felt the same way I did. They didn't see themselves in models either.

I can't remember exactly when it happened, but at some point I formed this really specific scene in my mind, and it would replay often. In it, a young girl kisses her parents goodbye, steps out the front door, then starts walking to school. On her way, she passes a massive billboard adorned with a stereotypically beautiful model — an image that's been retouched, perfected and curated to the extent that it doesn't even look like the model does in real life. The young girl sees it. She stops and she thinks, *That woman looks so perfect.*

The young girl keeps walking, and she passes another billboard with another retouched image. Later, at home, she reads a magazine filled with more photos of retouched models, and on TV she sees commercials with even more images of uniformly perfected people. All the models look the same. Everyone is the same — everyone, that is, except the young girl. *I don't look anything like any of those women,* she thinks. *I'm not beautiful or perfect like they are. There must be something wrong with me.*

Every time I saw this young girl in my mind, I felt so concerned for her. I worried for her sense of self-worth, for her confidence, for her mental health. I couldn't help but think of the day, not so far in the future, when she would be old enough to start making decisions about her own body — and how she might try to alter it to match the image of that 'perfect' model she'd been bombarded with, even though those perfections never actually existed in the first place. Perhaps this scene was a subconscious product of my own experience. That young girl could easily be little Jess on her way to school, feeling like her recently reconstructed body would never be enough in a world that curated such a narrow and prescriptive view of happiness and beauty.

I knew things needed to change, but I didn't quite know *how*. What I really wanted was to find a way to show that young girl that her differences were okay, because everyone is different. I wanted to find a way to tell her she was enough, that she was okay exactly how she was. I wanted the world to stop making her question her self-worth and her own beauty. In fact, I wanted the world to stop placing importance on beauty at all.

What I really wanted was to find a way to show that young girl that her differences were okay, because everyone is different. I wanted to find a way to tell her she was enough, that she was okay exactly how she was.

Then, one day, I put that scene on pause. *What if I flipped it?* I thought. *What if that young girl walked past a different kind of image — one of someone like me? Someone living in a body that differed from what she was so used to seeing?* I wondered what it would mean if, instead of hiding or trying to erase our differences, we shared them. What if we showed them to the world? Would that change how the young girl felt? Would she feel like she was enough?

Another scene began to unfold in my mind: one where that young girl walks past a different kind of billboard, one showing a young woman proudly wearing her blade. It was a dream — and a far-fetched one, I knew — but I thought something like that could be a start. Something like that might bring the change we needed.

THE PHOTO SHOOT WITH Jono and Courtney was my first as a model, and it was a lot of fun. We went with a few different looks — some quite sporty and some more fashion-based — and when Jono sent me the images a few days later, I felt on top of the world. They were amazing. For the first time ever, I felt genuinely confident — and I looked it. In every shot, the blade was a prominent feature, and it had suddenly become my superpower. It looked so cool. It's like I'd found a piece of myself that I hadn't even known was missing.

In my favourite shot, I was standing facing the camera, wearing a black crop top and black high-waisted underwear. My hair was slicked back, and a coat covered most of my body but stopped just below my knee, showcasing my blade. At the time, I was on Instagram and occasionally posted photos with weird sepia filters and white borders, because apparently that was cool, but most of my followers were friends and family, or their friends. That's pretty much all I knew about the world of social media. I posted the photo and captioned it 'Limbitless' — a nod to the title of the thesis I'd completed the year before, in which I'd researched prosthetics in fashion. That caption embodied everything I felt my postgraduate study and the shoot with Jono and Courtney had been about.

A week or so later, I posted a couple more images I loved from the shoot. In both, I was wearing a white Nike singlet with the same black high-waisted undies. My hair was pulled back, and I sat on a ledge in a white studio, my right leg bent and my blade out straight. In one shot, I looked right down the barrel of the camera with a serious expression, and in the other I was smiling.

I captioned this post 'Breathe. Smile. & don't let anyone kill your vibe', then forgot about it.

THE FOLLOWING NIGHT, ONE of my best friends, Jesse, and I headed round to another friend's house with some takeaways. On the way, we somehow got talking about social media.

'You know people buy followers, eh?' Jesse said.

'No they don't,' I replied.

'They do,' he insisted.

'I don't believe you,' I said, and I meant it, which shows just how clueless I was about the world of social media.

'It's true. I could go and buy you a bunch of followers right now,' he said. 'And it would look like you have way more than you actually do. But it'd just be a bunch of bots and fake profiles and stuff.'

Jesse is just the kind of guy who would actually do something like that because he thought it was funny.

'If you ever buy me followers,' I said, 'I will never speak to you again.'

He laughed, but I was deadly serious. The idea of having followers was weird enough to me, but buying followers that weren't even real just so you could say you had them? That was even weirder.

I opened the app, and saw my notifications menu was filled with new comments and new followers. When I refreshed the screen, it refilled with a whole new batch. They just kept flooding in.

We got to our friend's house, and the conversation moved on. Later in the evening, after we'd eaten and were reaching the end of a movie, my phone started lighting up. I picked it up and had a look. All the notifications were from Instagram.

I opened the app, and saw my notifications menu was filled with new comments and new followers. When I refreshed the screen, it refilled with a whole new batch. They just kept flooding in.

I immediately turned on Jesse. 'What have you done?' I said furiously.

'What? Nothing!' he said.

'Really?' I glared at him. 'You didn't go and buy me followers?'

'No! I have no idea what you're talking about,' he said.

I showed him my phone.

'Holy shit,' he said, watching the notifications continue to roll in. 'Yeah, that's got nothing to do with me.'

It wasn't until we worked out that one of my photos from the shoot had been reposted on an account with over a million followers that I finally believed him. Soon, the same photo had been shared again on another account. All night, the notifications kept coming. I went to bed feeling pretty overwhelmed, but I told myself that it would have all blown over by the morning.

It hadn't.

By the time I left for work the next day, I had more than 10,000 followers — and counting.

4

Breaking out of boxes

Some people like to put things in boxes. They like to understand things as quickly and easily as possible. They like things to make sense — and that includes other people. But boxes are suffocating. They're the wrong shape for human beings. We just don't fit in them.

If someone else tries to put you in a box labelled 'normal' but you burst the whole thing wide open, that might cause them discomfort. They might see it as a challenge. They might want to force you to fit, to conform, but that's never going to work. And that boxing-in impulse? It's all on them.

You don't owe anyone an apology for defying their imaginary box. You don't have to apologise to someone who can't — or won't — expand their own narrow view of the world.

Let's stop putting each other in boxes. Let's stop trying to categorise one another. We are all human. We are all different. If we want to find true equality, across the board, we need to let go of the desire to box one another in.

FOR THE FIRST FEW years after my cancer treatment and having my leg amputated, I was pretty carefree. It never crossed my mind that I might be 'different'. I didn't take any notice of people staring at me, and I never felt sorry for myself. I was just happy to be where I was.

Then, around the age of thirteen, I hit a wall. Forcefully. *Smack.* It was honestly like I woke up one day and everything sank in. Things started to make sense in a way that I didn't want them to. It's like my childhood naivety had evaporated and I was suddenly seeing everything for what it really was. I had reached an age and a maturity where I began to fully comprehend the implications of everything I had been through. It was a lot. Not only was I having to adjust to a whole new body, but I was also dealing with the trauma of what I had seen and felt and experienced at such a young age. There was the physical pain I've already mentioned —

the blisters, the nerve pain, the calluses — but there was also the pain of coming to terms with the fact that there would forever be things I would have to do differently or not at all. For four years, I'd been acutely aware of the way my body felt. Learning to walk again will do that. It forces you to develop an above-average sense of physical self-awareness. I was conscious of every movement required to take first one step and then another — I knew every aspect of the way it felt, the pain it caused. But I had zero awareness of how my body looked in comparison to others' bodies. It just wasn't something I cared about.

That was when I suddenly refused to wear shorts any more. I didn't want anyone to see my prosthetic side. I let my fear of being different tell me I should hide away.

But, as soon as I hit my teens, I began to notice people staring when I walked down the street. For the first time, I started to feel self-conscious about the way I looked. As I grew, my body began to fill out, and my prosthetic side became thinner and thinner in comparison to my right leg, since my thigh (which was really a calf, remember) was never going to grow like the other thigh. I realised that, even when I wore long pants, the size difference was obvious because one side sat looser than the other. That was when I suddenly refused to wear shorts any more. I didn't want anyone to see my prosthetic side.

I let my fear of being different tell me I should hide away. Soon it ruled my life. I became obsessed with trying to make my legs look like they were both the same size. Each day, I would wake up and wrap multiple T-shirts and socks around my thigh-slash-calf, then secure everything in place with masking tape and a sports bandage. And, every night, in order to be able to remove my prosthetic leg, I would have to unravel the whole lot, only to get up and do it all over again the next day.

I stopped wanting to go out with family and friends. At the time, I didn't think anyone else noticed what I was doing. Then, one night when I was getting ready to go to a show a friend was performing in, I got so frustrated by how my leg looked that I completely broke down. My whole family was going to the show too, and they were waiting for me, but I just refused to go. Mum ended up staying home with me. I could tell she was upset too, although she understood. I guess she was sad to see that I was letting the way I looked hold me back. To this day, I don't remember what we talked about, but I do know that's when I realised my hiding away hadn't gone totally unnoticed.

I just saw myself as so far from normal. I felt so insecure. My body didn't look at all like the bodies I saw around me — not my friends', not my family's, not anyone's on TV.

The only time I saw bodies even close to my own was when I went to my monthly check-ins at the Limb Centre, but that felt so clinical and I couldn't really relate to the bodies of the other amputees. Even in that environment, when I took my leg off people would stare in confusion at my backwards foot. I felt alone. I felt trapped in a body I didn't want to be in.

My self-consciousness would rear its head in so many mundane everyday experiences — the sorts of things I could never have considered I'd miss doing, the sorts of things people with two legs so easily take for granted. Things like hitting the bottom of a staircase and realising you can't race up it as fast as your brain wants you to, or the ability to simply step out of the shower and stand on two feet. The ability to walk on tiles or wooden floors without socks or a grippy sole in case one drop of water sends you and your plastic foot straight to the ground. The ability to jump into the back of a car when your friends pick you up without stressing about whether your leg will fit inside or not — which, nine times out of ten, it doesn't, meaning you have to either prop it at an uncomfortable angle or awkwardly get everyone to shuffle seats so you can sit up front. The ability to go through the day without having to think about how you're going to move your body from A to B. The ability to just decide, on the spur of the moment, while you're walking along the beach to run into the ocean, without first having to change into your 'swim leg'. The ability to run for shelter when a rainstorm comes bucketing down. The ability to run at all.

Every morning, I would wake up wishing I wasn't living in the body I had. I wasn't sure how I would get through the day, but I knew I didn't have a choice. And, during the day, I was mostly okay. Sometimes, little things would trigger me at school and I would get down. When I first thought about trying out for netball teams at high school, for instance, I was initially reluctant for one reason: I was worried about how my leg would look in a short netball skirt. As my friends' school skirts progressively got shorter, mine just kept getting longer. I'd sweat through the hot, humid Auckland summers in long pants or long denim shorts that went below my knee. If Mum was picking me up from school and I knew we'd have to go and run errands, I'd ask her to bring trackpants so I could change out of my school skirt as soon as possible. I always told her it was because I was cold — clearly, she saw straight through that, but she still brought the trackpants for me every time without saying anything. I remember being at family social gatherings and always standing slightly away from everyone just so I could hide my leg behind the nearest side table or pot plant.

On the outside, I was confident. If anyone ever asked about what I'd been through or what happened to my leg, I would happily tell them — but I wouldn't show them. It

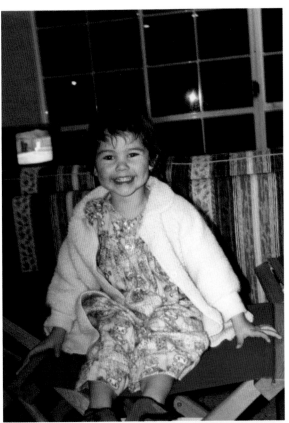

Left
Me at two years old, with my
trademark beaming smile.

Below
Taking part in a ballet
recital at age seven.

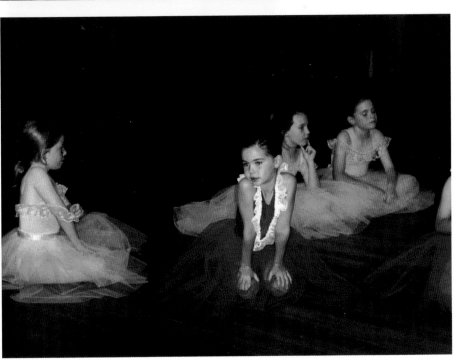

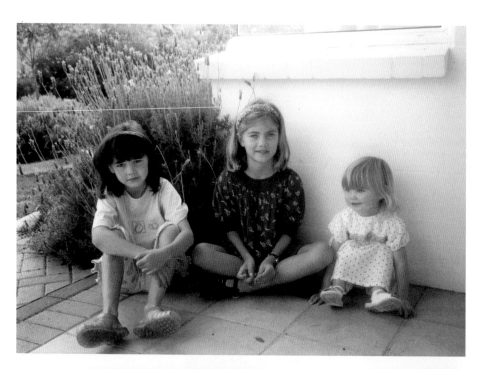

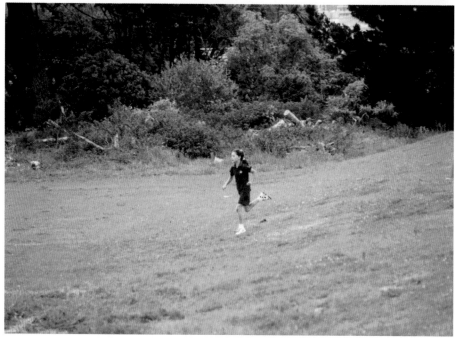

Top
Posing for a photo at our family home in
Albany with my sisters, Abby (centre) and
Sophie-Rose (right).

Bottom
Competing in a school
cross-country race at the age of eight.
Running was my thing as a kid.

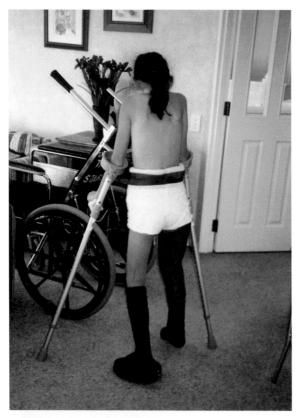

Left
Getting to grips with my
crutches and hip spica
(plaster cast) after breaking
my femur in March 2001.

Below
My sisters checking out my
hip spica and wheelchair
outside our house in Albany.

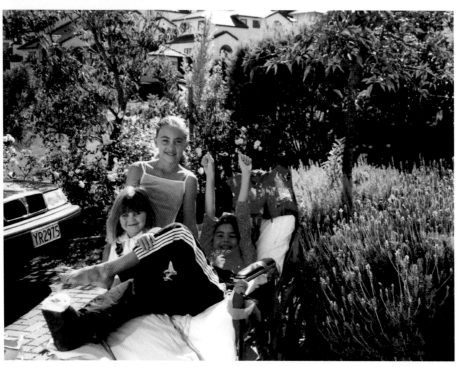

Right
With my mum, Debby, at
a hospital check-up before
I started chemotherapy in
July 2001.

Below
Still smiling through
the chemo.

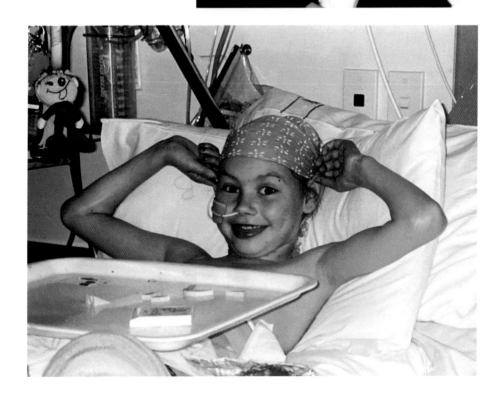

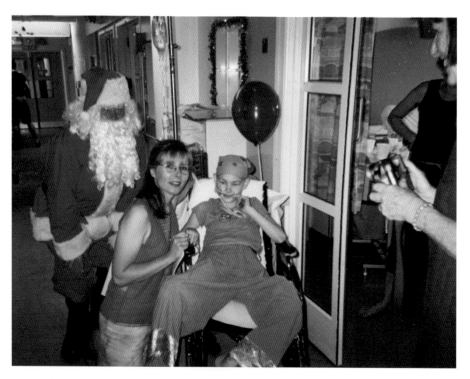

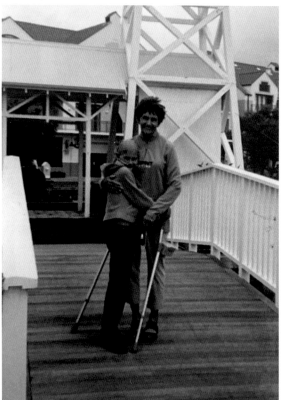

Above
Meeting entertainer Suzy Cato in hospital while receiving chemotherapy. Years later, we would appear together in the same season of *Dancing with the Stars*.

Left
With Nana Jan, exploring the world outside the hospital on a day off from treatment.

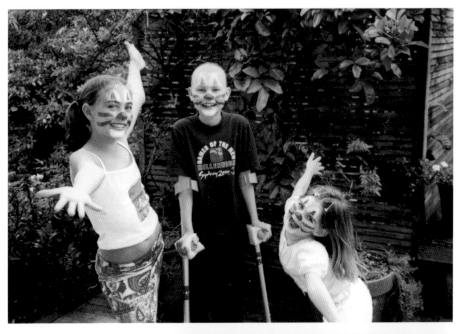

Above
Having fun with my sisters at home during a gap between chemo treatments.

Right
Meeting a friend's puppy at home in Albany. Later, Mum and Dad let me get my own dog to celebrate finishing chemo and getting out of hospital.

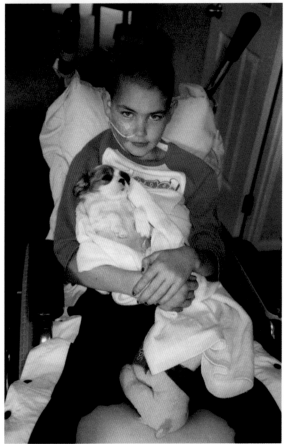

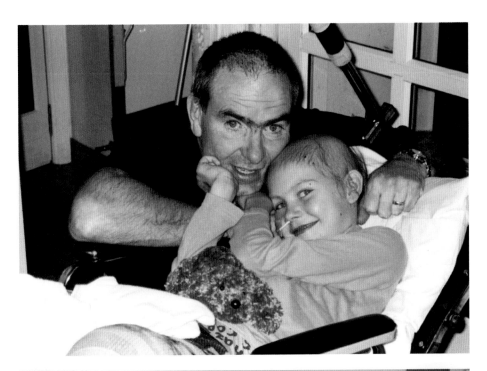

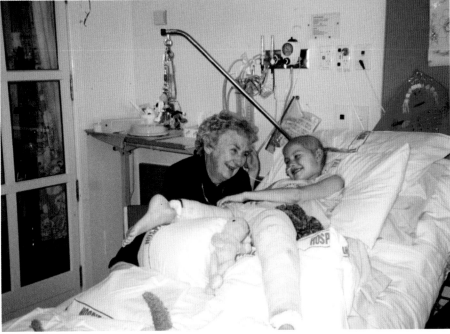

Top
My dad, Jim, can always reassure me
with his gentle bedside manner.

Bottom
Having a laugh with Grandma Ann
while recovering from my
rotationplasty surgery.

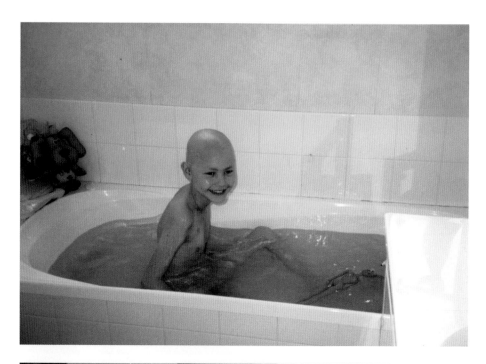

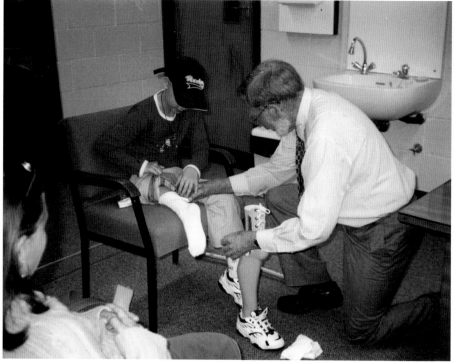

Top
My first bath following the
amputation and rotationplasty.

Bottom
At the Limb Centre, getting fitted
with my first prosthetic leg.

felt easier to hide it away, and soon it just became what I did. Now, I wonder who I was hiding it from. Was it from the judgement of the world around me or was I actually just hiding it from myself? Was I trying to avoid having to see it all the time and be reminded of every single way my new body was different? It was never a conscious decision, more something that seemed the easiest way for me to try to move on. It was by far the easiest way for me to try to blend in and to fit into this idea of 'normal' that I'd come to believe existed.

On the outside, I was confident. If anyone ever asked about what I'd been through or what happened to my leg, I would happily tell them — but I wouldn't show them. It felt easier to hide it away, and soon it just became what I did.

When it came to netball, though, hiding my legs under long pants just wasn't going to be an option. So, in order to step out onto the court in the skirt I had to wear, I got myself a black knee brace that I would strap on above my prosthetic in the hope that it would look like I had a sprained knee. I also got a netball skirt that was three sizes too big, so that it would hide as much of my upper leg as possible. It was so enormous I had to pull the drawstring in all the way to stop it from falling down. My intense desire to play sports ultimately overcame my self-consciousness, forcing me to find a way to get on with it, but I wasn't comfortable in my body at all.

My insecurities controlled my life. It was no longer good enough that I had a life to live. I can't even count the number of times I refused to go somewhere because I couldn't wear high heels, or because I didn't like the way my leg looked in my dress, or because I was self-conscious of the way my prosthetic thigh fell down and caused my pants to bunch up. I remember getting ready for a birthday party with some friends once, and suddenly feeling so low about myself that I made an excuse to leave. I don't know who I was trying to impress. All I can say is that I felt, at the time, that it was so important to be the same as everyone else. I just wanted to fit this image of perfection, of what was 'normal', that I believed existed.

Not many people would have known how much I was struggling, though. I didn't share what I was going through with anyone else. It just seemed easier to deal with it all quietly, in my own head. I never wanted to tell Mum and Dad about the battles I was fighting, because I didn't want them to feel any more pain on my behalf. That's just how I am. I've always found it's easiest to ride the wave, to figure things out on my own. I never really felt like anyone could fully relate to what I was going through, so instead of trying to make people understand, I learnt to just sit with it. Now I know that bottling things up like that isn't necessarily the best and I probably should have talked to my parents in particular. But they also knew — they kept a much closer eye on me back then than I ever realised. I believe it's good to talk, to get things out, to let your community in on the battles you're fighting, and I've become so much better at seeking help when I need it. But I didn't know all that back then.

Some evenings I would get so angry with my leg that I'd hurl it across my bedroom and it would hit the wall with a satisfying *thud*.

It was at night, when the world got a little quieter, that all these feelings became much harder to avoid. Some evenings I would get so angry with my leg that I'd hurl it across my bedroom and it would hit the wall with a satisfying *thud*. That's one good thing about prosthetic legs — they make great anger-management tools.

I obviously put mine to good use in that sense, because one day it started making a strange clicking noise. I took it to the Limb Centre, only for Mum to get a voicemail a few days later: 'Hi, Debby. Just letting you know Jess has broken her leg . . .' After a brief panic, Mum established that they were talking about my carbon-fibre leg, *not* the one made of flesh and bone, and all was okay after a quick screw replacement. Among the hardships, these moments of comic relief were definitely welcome. Sometimes there's nothing you can do but laugh.

It was a really difficult time, but throughout it all I tried to remind myself that it was just a season. I held on to the fact that it would pass, that it was just another part of my journey, that I'd get through somehow. Even so, I cried myself to sleep more often than not. I'd work myself up into complete hysterics, quietly mumbling the words 'Why me?' over and over again until I finally passed out from exhaustion.

The next morning, the tears would have crusted around my eyes, but I'd wash them off, strap my leg on and tell myself, 'You've got this.'

WHEN I WAS ABOUT fourteen, Dad — clearly noticing how much of my life I was missing out on because of my insecurities about my thigh — came up with a plan. He started asking around and somehow, by going from one contact to another, he managed to get himself an introduction to Sir Richard Taylor. Yes, *the* Richard Taylor, founder and creative director of Weta Workshop, famous for the four Academy Awards he won for his work on the Lord of the Rings trilogy.

'I've been speaking to Richard,' he told me (they were on

first-name basis by this point), 'about building you a thigh.'

Usually, Weta's busy creating enormous, lifelike monsters and elaborate props for movies. Dad figured that meant they could surely build one little thigh. So he went ahead and asked. That's Jim Quinn for you: well connected and not afraid to think outside of the box. Amazingly, Richard agreed to help.

So, before I knew it, Dad and I were on a plane down to Wellington. When we got to Weta Workshop, the team there took plaster moulds of both legs, and used those to create another mould for building my new thigh. For months, they worked on it, sending prototypes back and forth to test and then modify, until I eventually had a brand-new prosthetic thigh. It was made out of foam and Lycra, and sat over the top of my current prosthetic, meaning it filled out my jeans — and slowly helped me build the confidence I'd lost.

This hasn't been without its stresses. To begin with, my thigh would only last about three months, as the foam would break down, so I'd get a new one in the mail several times a year. Over time, I was able to make each thigh last a bit longer, but I eventually had to get a new mould made. As my body grew and changed, that meant my thigh needed to change too. What's more, at different stages, manufacturing has stopped and started. The technology used to create these things changes every time, so it's never straightforward. But nothing is ever without its challenges, and none of that takes away what the thigh has given me.

I often wonder how I would feel about my body had it not been for prosthetics like this. Am I only accepting being different within the realm of the illusion I have created?

To this day, it remains a constant part of my life. I don't go a day without wearing it. I often wonder how I would feel about my body had it not been for prosthetics like this. It changed my life. As my career has developed and I've become vocal about normalising different, I have asked myself if I only feel this way because of the privilege I had in accessing a prosthetic like this. Am I only accepting being different within the realm of the illusion I have created? Honestly, I don't have an answer to that, and I admit I've felt like an imposter time and time again.

In order to test whether I'm still okay in this body of mine, without all of its additions, I'll sometimes force myself to spend time without my thigh on. There are a couple of things I have realised from doing this. The first is that, while the thigh began as a purely cosmetic solution for an insecure teen, it's now basically a physical necessity. Without it on, life is a struggle. My pants bunch up and get caught in the hinges of my prosthetic leg when I walk or move. It's not comfortable to cross my legs or sit without a thigh there to fill the gap between me and the seat or my good thigh and my prosthetic. So there's that. There's also the fact that the thigh has helped me get to where I am. It's helped me bridge the gap between lost little fourteen-year-old Jess and me today — a person who can walk around confidently with a blade for a leg and not care who shoots looks my way.

ONE BEAUTIFUL SUMMER'S AFTERNOON in my second-to-last year of high school, I was at a friend's house, hanging out beside her pool. There was a small group of us there, all close friends, and everyone except me was wearing shorts or skirts or togs. I was wearing long pants, and by this time I was seventeen — meaning I'd spent eight long years sweating through summer days just like this one. It had become such a habit that I didn't think anything of it.

Then the friend whose house we were at said, 'Jess, you must be so hot in those pants! Do you want to borrow some shorts?'

She said it so casually that I don't think she'd even really thought about why I might be so overdressed on such a scorching day. And, since she didn't make a big deal of it, I found myself thinking, *Why not?*

'Yeah, okay,' I said. 'That'd be awesome.'

So we went up to her room, where she got me out a pair of shorts and left so I could get changed.

'Meet ya back at the pool,' she yelled as she shut the door behind her.

I don't know whether she ever realised just how much my life changed that day.

I put those shorts on and began to feel not only much cooler, but also like I'd suddenly shed a massive burden. It's like I was no longer holding on to something that I'd been carrying around with me for far too long.

I realised that the things you worry about often aren't even things that anyone else would ever notice. It's so easy to let your insecurities become much bigger than they ever need to be.

I made my way back out to the pool, expecting it to be just as big a deal to my friends as it was to me. But no one reacted at all. I just slipped back in, and we continued with whatever we were talking about, as though nothing had changed.

That was such a pivotal moment in my life. I realised that the things you worry about often aren't even things that anyone else would ever notice. It's so easy to let your insecurities become much bigger than they ever need to be.

After that day, I never looked back. I kept wearing shorts whenever I felt like it.

I often think about the little high-fives my parents must have been giving each other behind my back when they saw I was starting to shed some of those insecurities and becoming happier in my own skin. I know it must have been just as pivotal for them to see me slowly but surely coming to terms with the things that make me different.

I AM, QUITE LITERALLY, a walking miracle. Here I am, still standing, in a body that has been completely restructured so that I could survive an aggressive cancer. Every time I remember this, it makes almost no sense in my brain. It's truly incredible.

And yet, I spent those short few years as a teenager doing what way too many of us do: I reduced my body to aesthetics. Whenever I caught a glance of my body in the mirror, I would pull it apart. I was so afraid of other people's critical eyes that I hid my body away. But it turned out that the only critical eyes were my own. The only person standing in the way of my miraculous body doing all it could was me.

I so desperately wanted two legs, because that's what all my friends had. I wanted to be able to do everything they were doing. I thought they were 'normal', and that's what I wanted too. But I was so busy comparing myself to others that I failed to see the gifts I'd been given. I could only see the exterior, and that meant I missed what I held inside: the gift of survival, of going through the sort of experience that had forced me to see the world in a whole new light, and of courage, bravery and strength. None of these traits had *anything* to do with my appearance.

You may think the grass is greener for someone else, but what if that's because it's raining on them? You might be so caught up wondering why your grass isn't green that you've missed the sun shining above you.

Teenage Jess was not alone in this oversight. Way too many of us spend so much time comparing ourselves to friends, colleagues, siblings and strangers that we forget the miracle we are living in. We become so focused on the lives of others that we forget about our own.

You may think the grass is greener for someone else, but what if that's because it's raining on them? You might be so caught up wondering why your grass isn't green that you've missed the sun shining above you. Maybe your grass will be green if you take the time to water it? Maybe that other person's grass isn't even real grass?

Ultimately, I'm grateful that I went through everything I did at such a young age. I was forced to confront my insecurities before they took over my whole life. I had to accept that comparing myself to others just wasn't going to work — my body and my experiences were so unique it was pretty much impossible to match them to anyone else's. That's not to say I don't still have days when I judge myself harshly or want to throw in the towel. I'd love to wake up in the morning and walk (not crawl) to the shower, slip into a nice heeled shoe (not the flattest sneaker I can find), walk (not limp) up the stairs, and step outside my house without pain, discomfort or challenge. But I'm grateful to live in a body that has taught me so much. I'm grateful for this body — even on the days when it doesn't work in the way I'd like it to — simply because it's mine. I no longer try to change the things I have no control over. Instead, I'm determined to change the images on the billboards. I want that young girl in my mind to see more than one narrow view of the world. I want her to know that she is enough. I want to dismantle this idea of 'normal', to burn those boxes, to embrace difference.

I used to think it was so unfair that I didn't get to keep the body I was born in. Just as I was starting to understand its abilities, to love them, parts of it were taken from me. But then it dawned on me that none of us get to keep the body we were born in. We are constantly evolving, changing, growing. We all bear scars we didn't have when we arrived on this planet, and those scars are part of our stories. It still breaks my heart to think of the years I spent beating myself up for having one leg, as if it was something I asked for. How much life did I miss out on living during that time? Who might I have met at those events I never attended? How many people did I walk right past without realising they felt every bit as different and alone as I did? Imagine if I had kept living like that — all the friends I might have missed out on meeting, all the opportunities that would have remained hidden to me, all because I was hiding myself.

I wish more than anything that I could go back and talk to teenage Jess about all of this. Here's what I would say:

> Yes, your body does differ from the bodies of others, but you are not alone in that. Although your differences are unique, you are not unique in having differences. That's one thing we all have in common.
>
> I am so sorry your body doesn't match the idea of 'normal' the world has fed you, but know this: your differences are your superpower. One day you will realise this, and on that day you will be more grateful for your differences than you could ever have imagined possible.
>
> Please don't lose any more life than you already have by worrying about this body you're in. This body is a miracle. It saved you. And

I know for sure that everyone who loves you, everyone who helped you fight so hard for this life, would be devastated to learn you're wishing away the thing that saved you. And whenever it feels unfair, be patient. I promise you, the lesson will come if you're open to accepting it.

There's a big world out there, and it needs bodies like yours. Bodies so unique that they remind others that being different is more than okay. Bodies that remind us that 'normal' isn't real, and it never was.

This world is yours for the taking, Jess! Nothing can hold you back but the walls of your own mind. So let your hair down, worry less, feel free more. Don't be held down or held back by the things that make you different.

You are enough. You are *more* than enough, exactly as you are. Stop trying to fit into a box that was never built for you.

You're so much bigger than that.

THE WEEKS FOLLOWING THAT Instagram post going viral were a complete whirlwind. All of a sudden, I was in the spotlight. Articles about the photo shoot Jono, Courtney and I had done for fun started popping up, calling me a model, all over international news websites.

'Stunning model is out to prove confidence is more beautiful than perfection,' declared the *Huffington Post*, while the *Daily Mail* proclaimed, 'Woman, 23, who lost her leg to bone cancer lands job as a model after posting pictures with her prosthetic limb on Instagram.' I had local news shows calling me at work to request interviews, and my follower count on Instagram just kept growing and growing. Within a few months, it had reached more than 70,000. Almost overnight, I'd been propelled from clueless about social media to what people were then just beginning to call an 'influencer' (a term I'm still not the biggest fan of).

It all happened so quickly that I never really had much time to think about how many people I was sharing my life with. And the messages I started receiving from people all around the world, from all walks of life, were incredible. These people — total strangers — were reaching out to tell me they found comfort in my story. It was amazing, and it just encouraged me to share more.

As I've said, I was always open with people about how I'd lost my leg. I had to be — I wore that particular vulnerability on the outside. I might have been able to downplay it with a prosthetic that looked like my other leg, by hiding it under long pants or behind pieces of furniture, but it was pretty obvious as soon as someone noticed it. But I never, ever let anyone see what my amputated leg really looked like.

I worried that boys wouldn't find me attractive, or that I'd get sympathy I didn't want. I accepted that I couldn't avoid sharing some of my vulnerabilities, but I wouldn't share anything more than I had to. One of my greatest insecurities was (and, I admit, still sometimes is) the point where my butt meets my prosthetic. Since my surgeon had to cut so high into my thigh to get rid of the cancer, I don't have a seamless transition from butt to flesh-and-bone thigh. I used to wish they'd been able to salvage the top of my thigh so it would look nicer, but that simply wasn't an option.

The more I told of my story, the more others wanted to tell me theirs. I began to see how, far from being a weakness, vulnerability can actually be powerful. It's scary to share your insecurities, but when you do so you give others permission to be vulnerable too.

I never used to tell anyone any of that, let alone show them. But then I started to share these sorts of stories on Instagram, and something incredible happened — something I hadn't anticipated. The more I told of my story, the more others wanted to tell me theirs. I began to see how, far from being a weakness, vulnerability can actually be powerful. It's scary to share your insecurities, but when you do so you give others permission to be vulnerable too. You create a space where people feel it's safe to open up. You start to realise just how many of us feel insecure about something.

So I started opening up more. I spoke about what I'd been through, what I worried about, what mattered to me, what empowered me. I tried to be honest about my relationship with my body, explaining that, while I'm never going to love the way it looks, I've got a stupid amount of love for the life and the abilities and lessons it's given me. I used my own experiences to encourage others to let go of trying to be anything other than themselves. Sure, sometimes my captions had more cheese than a cheese platter, but I was okay with that. I felt I'd finally been given an opportunity to tell that young girl walking past the billboard that she was enough, and I wasn't going to let it pass me by.

I began to get requests from brands that wanted to combine my mission with theirs, and was soon regularly booked for photo shoots and other partnerships. I also started a blog and began to do a bit of public speaking. As I got busier and busier, I had to take more and more leave from my day job. It soon became such a juggle that I had to make a decision: keep working in the field I'd studied so hard towards and loved, or leave it to pursue this new but uncharted opportunity that had suddenly opened up to me. It wasn't an easy choice to make, but I couldn't pass up the chance I'd been offered to use my story for good.

That meant leaving a place of security for a world I didn't really understand. There was a lot of uncertainty. I struggled a lot — and still do — with the idea that my new line of work didn't have a clear job title. Now, I think of it as telling my story on many different platforms, which is still a bit strange to wrap your head around. I can safely say I never imagined this might be the path I took, but everything that has come from it has had a much more enormous effect than I ever could have dreamt. It feels like what I was called to do.

AT THE SAME TIME as this new career path was taking shape, I was also right in the thick of training towards my ten-kilometre running goal.

I admit now that when I first set that goal, I didn't really know how far ten kilometres actually was. It just seemed like a good distance to be able to run. A nice round number. Something ambitious.

I began posting regularly about that journey and all the work I was putting in. I'd asked around for someone who could help me with my running training, and was put in touch with a guy who went by the name of Coach Sunz. I knew as soon as I met him that he was exactly the person I needed in my life: an Energizer Bunny full of running knowledge and experience. I started training with Sunz five or six days a week, often twice a day. We worked on everything: my stability, my mobility, my gait, my strength. Before long, I was jogging up and down the gym each day.

I also began to train with a good friend of mine, Lydia O'Donnell, who is a competitive runner. I still remember our first session together. It was the middle of 2016 by that point, and we'd arranged to meet at the track I had raced on as a kid, before I got cancer and was just starting to run competitively. I sat down on the side of the track and, as I removed my everyday prosthetic and replaced it with my blade, I looked out over the dewy grass. It glinted in the early-morning sun, the faintest mist hovering just above it. I was overcome with this incredibly strong sense of nostalgia, tinged with something I find it hard to put my finger on. The last time I'd run here, I'd been eight years old, had two legs and didn't have the faintest idea of the bomb that was about to go off in my young life. I couldn't help but think about how much my life had changed between then and now. How much I had changed.

I've had a few of these moments in my life, times when I feel this overwhelming sense of nostalgia or déjà vu. It's this sense of knowing I have been somewhere before, but in another life. It happens when I can't fully grasp a memory — it's dangling in front of me, but I can't fully jump into that body. To be honest, it's more like recalling a dream than a memory. But it *is* a memory: I'm remembering moments from my 'old' life, a life that doesn't feel like my own, a life where I had two legs. In these moments, I see how naive I was back then — not just to what the future held for me, but also to how strong I could be when the world demanded it.

That day on the track with Lydia, I managed to run a full lap. I had to stop and gather myself more than once. I felt like I might fall on my face more than once. But I did it: I ran 400 metres, every step of the way.

If I looked back over my life and mapped all the highs and lows, it was a bit like the line measuring a healthy heartbeat on a monitor: up and down, up and down, over and over.

I was that much closer to my goal of running ten kilometres by the end of the year. Just 9600 metres to go. To some, that might have seemed an insurmountable task, but to me? It was just another mountain.

By this point, I'd scaled enough peaks to know I was capable of taking on even the scariest ones. If I looked back over my life and mapped all the highs and lows, it was a bit like the line measuring a healthy heartbeat on a monitor: up and down, up and down, over and over. And, at every low point, I could hear myself saying, 'One day or day one, Jess? You decide.' That's another mantra I have. It's what comes to mind every time I doubt myself, every time I want to give up. It's how I remind myself that, if I want to get to the top of a mountain, the only person who's going to be able to make that happen is me.

So I pick myself up and say, 'Day one.'

5

Super-abled

Failure and success aren't black and white. There's no such thing as 'Did you fail?' or 'Did you succeed?' It's simply 'How and why did you get here?'

For a while, I was so tunnel-visioned about my goals that I couldn't see any of the other lessons I was being taught. I lost sight of where I was going, because I got stubborn about sticking to a side path. I had to sit back and take a better look around to understand it's never just about one particular goal, but about where you're going and how you're getting there. Once I realised that, everything made so much more sense.

Life is a journey. It's about learning and growing and figuring out who you are, who you want to be. If something isn't working for you or doesn't feel right, you're allowed to pivot. You can change your goal, adjust your direction. It's important to remember there's a bigger picture.

It's hard to let go of something you've told yourself — and others — you'll do, but sometimes it's necessary. That's how you'll learn that you really can do anything you set your mind to. If there's a will, there's always a way.

IF I WAS ASKED, I would say that I am a pretty lucky human. That might cause some people to raise their eyebrows, given the curveballs life has thrown me, but I *am* lucky. I was born into a life full of opportunity and love. I got to learn early just how quickly your world can change, just how precious life is and just how hard you can fight when you have to.

Sure, the experiences that taught me those lessons aren't something I would wish on anyone, but I'm still grateful for them. I know that this life can be taken from you at any second, so I don't wait to do things. I don't sit around hoping someone else will come along and build my dreams for me. I know I can fight anything life dishes out, and that's a strength I could never give up.

For a short time, while I was a teenager, 25 October was a date I dreaded. It used to be a sad day for me, a day when

I'd ask, 'Why me?' Now, it's a day I celebrate. It might be the day I lost my leg, the day my life got turned upside down and inside out, but it's also a day when I was incredibly lucky. That day, I kicked cancer's butt. I got to live.

That doesn't mean it was smooth sailing from that point. In fact, things only got harder and scarier after that. But I've found that's often the way with luck. Sometimes, it's when you come out of the scariest situations imaginable that you learn just how lucky you are.

Recently, Dad told me a story I'd never heard that illustrates this in the starkest terms. Shortly after I had my rotationplasty surgery, I was put back on the ward. Remember the goal was to eliminate the cancer completely, to make sure I never had to walk back into that hospital again, so no one was taking any chances. My tiny, reconfigured body began yet another gruelling round of chemotherapy. Right from the start, that had always been the plan. When I turned nine on 17 November 2001, just a couple of weeks later, I was a husk of the child I'd been on my previous birthday. I was still smiling, but I weighed just eighteen kilograms and the hair that had fallen out during my pre-surgery chemo and just started to grow back in uneven patches was soon falling out all over again.

For the most part, my chemo schedule rotated week on, week off, and if there were no complications I spent the in-between weeks at home instead of in the hospital. My doctors had arranged the dates so that I could be at home with my family for Christmas in 2001, but things didn't go according to plan. Late one night a few days before Christmas, my temperature spiked dramatically and my parents raced me back into hospital. After everything it had been through over the previous months, my body was so weak. My immune system was battling. As Dad put it when he was telling me this story, to me it was just another crap day in a long line of crap days, but what he and Mum saw was their little girl looking the worst she ever had. To them, it was clear I was barely holding on. They were really scared. Dad said it was the one time when he wondered, seriously, whether I was going to make it.

We arrived on the ward at the same time as another family with a young boy I'd met while I was in for chemo. He was fighting the same cancer I was, and also had a scarily high fever. He looked awful — worse than I'd ever seen him. We'd both reached the pit of our illnesses.

The two of us were admitted to hospital, and my doctors did everything they could. Somehow, I managed to sleep through the night, allowing the antibiotics that were pumped into my frail body to do their job.

The next morning, I woke up.

That young boy didn't.

It was when I first heard this story that it really hit home. I had always known things had been tough, that there had been times when a full stop hovered over me, waiting to end my story, but I had never properly grasped just how close it got. I almost died that night.

I was still in hospital when Christmas Day rolled around. Dad had stayed overnight with me, but Mum, my sisters, my aunty Shelly and Nana (Mum's mum) were at home when I woke up. Nana took a video of them that morning, and it's strange to see what my sisters went through — there's the usual sneaking around trying to work out what Santa has left, before Mum sits down with Abby and Soph to softly explain, 'It's time to pack up all the presents so we can take them in to Jessica at the hospital.' Life was so far from normal.

It's amazing how vividly I remember the moment my sisters rushed into my hospital room, given I was drifting in and out of consciousness, but I can still see them so clearly. They were bursting with excitement to see me, and to open our presents. Dad tried to sit me up so I could join in with them, but I was so weak, my lips cracked and dry, that I just had no interest whatsoever. Instead, I watched from a distance while Abby and Sophie joyously opened their gifts. I felt like I was floating above everything.

I stayed in hospital until just after New Year and then, at last, by some sort of miracle, I was well enough to be sent home. I simply cannot imagine what it was like for my parents to see their child in that state. There were countless times throughout that year (and the years to come) when I would start crying and Mum would say, 'I just wish I could swap places with you,' and Dad would say, 'If I had a magic wand I would make it all go away.' I can still hear it. You could see in their eyes that they meant every word.

By the time I was nine I'd experienced more death than I have in my whole life since. I'd make new friends in the hospital playroom who I'd see day after day, only to suddenly never see them ever again. One morning, the sister of a one-year-old patient came in and told me, 'My baby brother has gone to sleep forever.'

It's one thing to go through cancer, but it's another thing to survive. Everything I experienced during that time will stay with me. It's what reminds me every day of just how lucky I am. I will never know why I got to survive that night and that young boy didn't, but I'll forever be grateful for the second chance life gave me.

I believe that we all get taught the lessons we need in different ways and at different times. We can look at the people around us and compare our lives with theirs, and we can think that they have it easy because they're not facing the same hardships we are, but who are we to say their lesson isn't still on its way — or that they haven't already faced it? Or that what they've been through doesn't feel as big to them as our hardships do to us? Lots of us get caught in the trap of feeling frustration or sadness or anger towards our own experiences simply because we think we're worse off than others, but comparing our lives with others' just isn't a healthy way to live. I prefer to see my luck where it lies. Maybe I am no luckier than the next person, but I do know how to spot the strikes of magic. And I also truly believe that you never know what worse luck your bad luck might be saving you from.

Maybe I am no luckier than the next person, but I do know how to spot the strikes of magic.

Perspective is a beautiful thing.

Was I unlucky the day I broke my leg standing on that soccer ball? Or was I incredibly lucky, because that's what eventually led to the discovery of the danger that lay hidden beneath my skin?

Am I unlucky because I had a body part removed, relocated and reattached? Or am I incredibly lucky that such an advanced surgery was an option for me, simply because of the country I was born in?

Was I unlucky because I spent Christmas 2001 in hospital, teetering between life and death? Or am I lucky to have lived to see so many more Christmases with my loved ones since?

How could I sit here and say I'm not lucky when there's

a family out there whose son was in hospital at the exact same time as me and they never got to see him grow up?

How can I say I'm not lucky.

AS MY PUBLIC PROFILE grew, I did more and more interviews with various kinds of media, and I sometimes got asked questions that took me by surprise. One time, in an interview for a magazine feature, I was asked, 'If you could change what you went through, would you?'

Without even second-guessing myself, I immediately replied, 'No.'

It was such a bold question, I wondered at first how the interviewer had even thought it was okay to ask. But it also brought me to the sudden realisation that all of the awful things I had experienced — all of the pain, the illness, the constant change and adversity — had been worth it. It was in that moment that I realised the bad had been completely outweighed by the good. I wouldn't be who I am today without everything I've been through.

Another time, on live TV, I got asked how I felt about the word 'disabled'. My response: 'There are people with two legs more disabled than me because of their attitude. Me? I'm super-abled.'

For a second I wondered whether I'd said the right thing. I worried people would take it the wrong way. But I've since given this a lot of thought and have spoken about it, and I stand by that statement. I still feel it's true.

Around that time, I'd come across a TED Talk by an incredible woman named Aimee Mullins. She's a model and actor, a record-breaking athlete and a double amputee, and she opened her talk by running through the thesaurus entries for the word 'disabled' — example synonyms included 'crippled', 'helpless', 'useless', 'wrecked' and so on, while the antonyms were 'healthy', 'strong' and 'capable'. Just think about that for a second. And imagine, like I do, nine-year-old Jess reading those adjectives then applying them to herself. What would that have told her about what she was capable of? About what she was worth?

If you break it down, the word disabled quite literally means a lack of ability. Sure, in some ways I definitely have that. I can't move in the same way as most of the people I know. But there are also things that I can do better than some people I know, not because of my differences, but simply because I am human. We all have different abilities: some of us are naturally good at maths, some of us are born with incredible singing voices, some of us are athletic. None of us are able to do everything perfectly. We're all better at some things and worse at others. So doesn't that just make us all *differently* abled? And why, then, should we pick out a small part of the population and call them *dis*abled?

So, while I believe there is no right or wrong way to

identify, I have never identified as disabled. Over the years, I've asked myself whether that's just another way of hiding my insecurities or vulnerabilities, but it's not that. I fully accept my differences, and I'm okay with them — a large part of my job now is talking about just that — but I don't want to be placed in a box because of them. I don't want to live under a label that limits me. I want to use words for myself that empower me, push me, lift me up. That's why I prefer to think of myself as differently abled. And, if someone asks, I might even say I'm super-abled. I mean, come on — I have a carbon-fibre spring for a foot, and I get to change my legs depending on what I'm doing. If that's not super-abled, what is?

I don't want anyone else to be put in a box either.

Words are powerful. You define you. Write your own story.

I'VE SPENT A SIGNIFICANT portion of my life trying to test the limits of my abilities, and the ten-kilometre goal was just one example of this.

I have never been able to pinpoint exactly why I seem to want to keep pushing myself so much. It might be that I'm subconsciously trying to prove to myself that I can do things that seem impossible, or maybe I'm just reluctant to completely relinquish the athletic child I was before I lost my leg. Perhaps I just really love a challenge. Most likely, it's a combination of all of the above.

I was prepared for the fact that running ten kilometres would be a difficult road. I knew it wasn't going to be easy and that I'd have to put in the hard yards, but there was one thing I wasn't prepared for at all: the toll it would take on my good leg. Since my rotationplasty, my left leg has been my saving grace. It's my safety net, and it's always been incredibly strong. If my prosthetic side ever feels sore, my weight will fully shift to the left side, often without me knowing it. I can't feel my right leg in the same way as my good leg — I get a bit of sensory feedback from my foot that's acting as my knee, but it's not the same — so I'm not able to tell whether I'm walking with an even amount of weight through each leg or not.

I rely on my left leg in a big way. For every trip, fall, loss of balance and bout of pain, it has been there for me. It's my saviour — and, since my brain has got so used to knowing that, it lets my body rely on my left leg more and more. That wasn't always the case, of course. When I first started learning to live in this body, my left leg had to adapt like the rest of me and I remember having issues with it for a few years. It was dealing with a lot: the growing pains most teenagers experience, as well as learning to be the steady base for my whole body. At times, the pain that sat mostly around my kneecap and upper thigh became too much and

I'd end up back at the hospital. I was, not surprisingly, pretty nervous about any kind of pain — I was well practised at bearing it, but the last time I'd been in ongoing pain I'd ended up being told I had cancer and had lost my leg. And the first five to ten years post-cancer are the scariest, with everyone fearing that anything unusual is a secondary cancer that's been overlooked. So every time my left leg flared up, my doctors would run all of the tests possible, but the pain was always put down to growth and overuse.

I told myself to ride the wave and manage the pain as best I could, and eventually my body would get used to its new job. I'd been given a taste of running, a taste of achieving something I'd never thought I would do, and I was determined to see it through.

Eventually, my left leg became invincible. And, because it's always been so strong, it was never my main focus in my running training. I did do some strength and rehab work with it, to help it adjust to the new movement and demands, but it turned out that wasn't enough. Around the middle of 2016, when I started training on the track with Lydia, my good calf began to hurt. Every time my leg hit the ground, I'd get a ping of pain. I did everything I could to support it — got a better shoe, strapped it, had regular physio.

Of course, I'd stopped growing physically by then, but I chose to see this as another type of growing pain: I was growing in terms of what I was expecting my body to be able to do. I told myself to ride the wave and manage the pain as best I could, and eventually my body would get used to its new job. I just had to stick with it. I'd been given a taste of running, a taste of achieving something I'd never thought I would do, and I was determined to see it through. 'You're not going to be defeated by a small hill,' I'd say to myself. 'Not when you've climbed a mountain to get here.'

My life revolved around training. It was my happy place. I was finally in an environment where I felt beyond capable, where I got to compete with only myself. I was still training twice a day, for up to three hours, but each session had become a mix of managing my left-calf pain while building the strength in my right leg. I would start at the gym at five in the morning, often doing my own training session without my blade. In the evenings, I would meet up with my coach and a group of other athletes who were all training towards their own goals. The pain didn't go away — in fact, it was getting worse — but I pushed that to the back of my mind. I loved every second of what I was doing. I wasn't going to stop.

But, as the months went on, the pain in my left calf increased. The pain that shot up it had turned from a ping to a high-powered blast of shattered glass.

'Jess, I think you might have shin splints,' my running coach said one day, but I persevered until I simply couldn't run any more. It was September by this point, and the most I had run in one go was 600 metres, but I was adamant I'd reach ten kilometres by the end of the year. Writing it down now, I realise it sounds delusional, but in my mind it made sense — all I had to do, I figured, was build my muscles up enough to put one foot in front of the other, and then the distance thing would just fall into place. Once you can run physically, then you can run far, right? I knew I already had the willpower to run for days. I just needed to nail the actual technique and physicality.

Under strict instructions from my running coach, I walked — with an even more obvious limp than what my prosthetic naturally gave me — into a sports specialist's clinic. As I took a seat in the waiting room, I felt a touch of excitement. I know that's a strange thing to say, but this waiting room had one major difference from all the others I'd spent so much time in: it wasn't full of sick people, but athletes. Everyone was here, like me, to recover from injuries they'd obtained through pushing themselves to the limit.

Once the specialist had ushered me into his office, I explained what had been going on. I must have said something like: 'So I lost my leg fifteen years ago, but recently I realised the only thing I still couldn't do was run. So I got a running blade made and spent nine months learning to run. Then, once I had run 50 metres, I decided I was going to run ten kilometres, but now my leg's a bit sore.'

I'm sure the specialist must have wondered if I was joking.

He assessed me and threw around terms like 'shin splints' and 'compartment syndrome', but I didn't pay that much attention. I'd had so much experience with doctors by then that I tended to take their 'orders' more as guidelines. I saw them as being a bit flexible, and I assumed I could hear what this specialist had to say . . . then carry on with my own plans. Nothing was going to stop me from achieving my goal. I'd already figured out what I was going to do: rest up for a bit, train as much of my body as I could while recovering, then I'd get back to it.

'You need crutches,' the specialist said, 'and you need to go and get an X-ray straight away.'

'Yeah, that's not going to work,' I said. 'I've got training this afternoon.'

But he'd obviously realised what he was up against, and just said firmly, 'You're not going to training today.'

Reluctantly, I sent a text message to my coach to cancel and hobbled out of the clinic on crutches as ordered. I hadn't been on crutches for fifteen years. The weird thing about it was that my legs had swapped places: now, the supporting leg was my prosthetic. It made getting around difficult, but I did what I could.

I was not at all happy about it.

A WEEK LATER, I went back to the specialist to review my X-ray. It turned out I'd been running on a stress fracture. And that pain I'd been feeling? It had been my bone slowly breaking due to the amount of stress it was under.

I left the clinic with strict instructions to rest and remain off my left leg, but I told myself it would be fine. I could still reach my goal of running ten kilometres in three months' time. How could I not? I'd said it out loud. I'd told everyone I was going to do it. More importantly, I'd told myself I was going to do it.

But, during the half-hour drive home, something changed in my mind. I got thinking about how important my left leg was to me. It had always been my rock, but I'd pushed it so far it had started to crack, literally. For months I'd ignored the pain and what it was trying to tell me — that my leg wasn't okay, that it needed a rest — because I was stubbornly fixated on achieving a specific goal. I wanted to be able to run ten kilometres so badly, but I'd never really stopped to ask myself why. Why *was* I holding so tightly to that goal?

I realised that, somewhere in my mind, I'd felt that if I could run again then I was no different from before I lost my leg. If I could run then I was 'capable'. I've never liked saying, 'No, I can't do that,' and running had always been the one thing in my life post-amputation that had challenged me on that point.

As I sat there in the car, my crutches on the passenger seat beside me, I realised it was time to let go of the ten-kilometre goal. If the price was my good leg, it simply wasn't worth it.

The only way I could have possibly failed was if I had never tried at all.

The minute that thought occurred to me, I felt so defeated. I felt like I had failed.

But then it dawned on me that the only way I could have possibly failed was if I had never tried at all. I could have easily stayed on the sidelines, using 'I can't run' as an excuse, but that's not what I did. I persevered, for years. Even after I'd tried as a kid to run at the local school with Dad, I hadn't given up. I'd come back as an adult to try again, ordering my running blade, spending nine months figuring out how to use it, setting myself an unimaginable task and spending many more months giving the goal everything I had.

I hadn't failed at all.

I had learnt to run.

Sure, it wasn't far — but it still counted. I had done something I'd never thought was possible. The distance had never actually been the point. The will to try in the first place was the point. I could hold my head high and say I had tried, and that was more than enough.

That short drive home was transformative. Somewhere in the space between feeling defeated and realising I hadn't failed, I discovered something I'd never quite given words to before: I can't do everything, but I *am* capable of giving anything a go.

That might sound like a bit of a contradiction, but it's true. The body I am in can't do everything. It can only handle so much. I *do* have limitations. But if there's a mountain I really want to climb, and if I set my mind to it, I will find a way to reach the peak. I might have to get there in my own way and in my own time. My peak may look different from others', but the only thing standing between me and what I want to achieve is my willingness to give it a go in some shape or form.

And success is there, so long as I'm willing to see it. It might not look like I thought it would, and it might not be the exact peak I first set my sights on, but it all comes down to what I choose to let myself believe. I could have kept persevering with running, pursuing that ten-kilometre goal. I could have let my fracture heal and got back to training, but at the end of the day the most important thing in the world to me wasn't being able to go for a ten-kilometre run. It was simply being able to live my life as well, as independently and with as much capability as possible. If that meant sacrificing running in order to care for my good leg, my only solid foundation, that's what I was going to do.

So I pretty much stopped running altogether.

It took a long time for my leg to heal, but after a number of months of rest and rehab I was able to start going back to the gym, and there I discovered just how much the blade had expanded my abilities. It wasn't just running I could do now. I got back into boxing, which I'd done a lot in the past, but with my blade on I found a whole new love for it, as I was suddenly able to move around the bag more easily and quickly. I could also do drills I'd never been able to do before learning to run, like shuttle runs and high knees. I took every opportunity for a light jog, even if it was just a quick toilet break or to grab my drink bottle. Running was still in my heart. There was, and always will be, something about it that just makes me feel good.

That was such a momentous time in my life. I learnt so much about myself and the body I live in, about success and failure, and about defining my own peaks — and the importance of changing them if necessary.

And, although I'd put my running goal to bed, that particular journey wasn't over yet. My blade was about to take me down a number of roads I could never possibly have predicted.

6

Perfectly imperfect

One thing we humans all have in common is that we're all different, yet we're living in a world that too often tells us that's wrong. Society offers just one cookie-cutter mould of perfection, and everyone who sits outside of it — which is to say, most of us — ends up feeling different and under-represented.

Well, now we've woken up to the world we're living in. We've decided that's not how we want things to be any more.

I'm here to add a different body into the mix. My hope is that I can show other young people, who are still busy growing up, that being different is, in fact, normal.

IF YOU'VE WATCHED MY journey unfold on social media, you know how raw and honest I am about what I tell and what I show. I talk openly about my life and my experiences, and I'm vocal about the need for wider representation and diversity in the way our world gets depicted. I'm grateful for the platform that social media has given me, because I know not everyone gets that opportunity — and I want to do everything I can with it to fight for a better world for all of us. Since I'm lucky to be surrounded by a community of people who want to hear what I have to say, I see it as part of my job to fight for everyone else who doesn't have that voice.

After my photo shoot with the blade went viral, my Instagram community just kept ballooning, and that carried on right throughout 2017. In the space of a little over a year, my world changed dramatically. The more people who read my posts, the more opportunities came my way — but I soon started to find social media and the new demands on my life overwhelming. I knew I needed to find someone to help me. When I got introduced to Brooke Howard-Smith, the CEO of an agency called WeAreTENZING, I was a bit nervous at first about getting management. I didn't want my story — something so personal to me — to be exploited, but as soon as Brooke explained that TENZING's mission is solely to help people with purpose, it instantly felt like a good fit. So that's how I ended up with a manager (yes, weird, it took me ages to get used to even saying that).

In the space of a little over a year, my world changed dramatically. The more people who read my posts, the more opportunities came my way — but I soon started to find social media and the new demands on my life overwhelming. I knew I needed to find someone to help me.

Together, Brooke and I did some planning sessions to explore how I could work with the brands that were approaching me on getting the message I wanted to share out into the world. From the get-go, I knew I wanted to do things that made a difference, and I definitely didn't want my Instagram page or the things I talked about to just become an advertising space. Telling my story had officially became my full-time job. While my life pre-2016 had been pretty private, now I was dealing with a constant flow of media, photo-shoot and brand-partnership requests. It was unexpected, to say the least. At times, when I took note of just how many people were watching and engaging with what I was doing, it felt unfamiliar and at times uncomfortable — but it felt right.

It was around this time that Instagram morphed from an app where people simply shared strange little snippets of their days into a highly curated feed of lives that none of us were actually living. We began connecting the dots between the snippets we consumed, and we used that to form an idea of how we believed people were spending their days. We forgot about the in-between moments, the ones that weren't captured, the things that we would have actually been able to relate to.

Where once upon a time we had mostly just seen pictures of people's pets or what they ate, now we began to be bombarded with bodies and stories that didn't actually exist. We were only being shown the best angles or carefully chosen shots. There were no stretch marks or cellulite or pimples or pores or bad hair days. We were only being shown images that — just like on those billboards — were so manufactured they didn't look like anything in the real world.

But this all happened so quickly that lots of us didn't

realise it straight away. We didn't realise we had begun to compare our lives to those we were consuming. We didn't realise that we'd started believing that these people were perfect and didn't experience hardship or insecurities. An app that was supposed to bring us together ended up making us feel even more separated from reality and from each other. We felt the distance widening between our own lives and what Instagram told us was 'normal', and we ended up every bit as insecure as we'd always been made to feel by older forms of media. But this was worse — this was in our pockets 24/7.

And, while we were all busy posting and absorbing this sort of content, we began to base our sense of self-worth on it. We valued our lives and our experiences according to how many people 'liked' our posts or followed us. Without even realising we were doing it, we began to equate attention with perfection. The more attention we got, the better we felt about ourselves. Comments telling us we were beautiful, worthy or living an enviable life provided the instant gratification we desperately sought to make ourselves feel like we were enough.

I am speaking in the most general terms here, of course. Every social media platform is different, and everyone chooses to express their life in a certain way. But there's no doubt about it: a lot of the forms of media that were supposed to make our lives more 'social' have had the opposite effect. We are connected, but only on a superficial level. And lots of us know more now about people we've never met than we do about our own friends and families.

When you care as much as I do about dismantling the boxes we put each other in, it's an interesting space to find yourself working in (probably the understatement of the century). I know insecurities, lack of self-confidence and body-image issues are beyond common, and that some people find comfort in knowing others aren't alone in those feelings. But me? It just makes me mad.

When you care as much as I do about dismantling the boxes we put each other in, the world of social media is an interesting space to find yourself working in.

Why are so many of us walking around hiding parts of ourselves away? I ask this because I really want you to ask yourself the same thing. I've spent years diving deep for the answer, and here's what I've come up with: too many of us have been told that the way we look is the only thing that matters, that being 'beautiful' is the currency we pay to exist. That's particularly true for women, although I know this definitely affects us all as humans. None of us are immune. But it's undeniable that the societal pressure on women to be a certain way runs many, many generations deep. Since before I existed, since before my mum existed, advertising has told women they must be nothing shy of perfect — but perfect within the limited box society maps out for them. 'You should look like this,' advertising whispers to us, before going on to tell us how to get the flawless skin or the tiny waist or the shiny hair we're meant to need. Setting aside the fact that it's ridiculous to suggest that flawless skin or a tiny waist or shiny hair could ever tell you anything about what a person's really like, the models we're shown as exemplars don't even exist. The images look nothing like the real women themselves. None of it exists. None of it is real. It is all made up.

So why do we give these messages so much airtime? Why do we let them distract us into spending so much time focusing on things that simply do not matter? Why do we skip out on occasions because we hate the way we look? Why do we spend our whole lives avoiding certain foods, afraid of what they'll do to our bodies? Why are we constantly trying to turn back time, to get back the bodies we used to live in?

We're so focused on the exterior, but that's just a shell. It's what houses your mind and your soul, but it can change at any moment. Your body may not change as drastically as mine did when I was eight, but I can promise you that it will change. As we age, we all gather scars and stretch marks. We grow, we change shape, and we barely have any control over most of it. If we stopped, just for a moment, we would learn to see these changes as miracles. They're what map our route through this thing called life.

Your exterior shouldn't get to have a say about what's going on inside you. After all, what good is a perfectly painted house if its contents aren't treasured? I want to see a shift away from this focus on the exterior. I want us to stop spending our lives trying to *look* a certain way and start concentrating on what we're going to *be*. Instead of spending our lives trying to be pretty or skinny or perfect, I want us to spend them trying to be kind, smart, loving, happy.

EARLY IN 2018, I flew to Sydney for a photo shoot. It was for an activewear brand, and it was one of the first times I was actually booked as a model. By that point, I'd done plenty of other shoots but most had gone alongside articles about my life.

I remember feeling so excited. A big international brand was flying me overseas so I could feature in their campaign, alongside three other models who were all different sizes and ethnicities. I felt like I was taking one step closer to normalising different. It was one of those moments when you realise you're actually living what was once just a far-fetched dream.

The team was incredible, as was the shoot. I was feeling at

my best and at a point where it seemed nothing could hold me down. The other models and I wore a variety of outfits that showed there's no right way to have a body, and we were photographed running up and down Bondi Beach at sunrise. That made the shoot really physically active — something a lot of people don't often realise about modelling. I wore my blade, but I had never attempted to run on sand with it before and I couldn't imagine how it was going to work. It's hard enough to run with two feet on the sand, let alone one foot and a curved metal spring. I was nervous about keeping up with the other models, especially since we were running up and down in front of the camera for a few hours, but I managed it. After a while, I started to feel my good leg giving in, but in true Jess style, I pushed through.

The next day, I was totally exhausted. During the flight back home to Auckland, my good leg was in so much pain, but that didn't bother me. I'd just done two things I'd once only dreamt of: running along a sandy beach and taking part in a photo shoot to shake the system.

Not long after getting home, I was sent the images. I loved them, and posted one that showed me running down the beach in shorts and a crop top with the caption:

> This image makes me so happy.
> Why? Because it's real. This is 100 per cent
> me. No photoshop, no trying to get the right

angle, just me exactly as I am, exactly as I should be. And beaming with smiles because I was so happy in that moment.

My biggest dream is to work with companies to normalise the use of real people in advertising and not by doing a big campaign that screams 'we're supporting real bodies' by adding one model with a slight curve.

No.

I want everyday people used, so that young people grow up seeing how everyday people look. It scares me that what they see is so filtered and photoshopped that they believe that's real.

I want kids to grow up knowing that their imperfections are what's real. That it's normal for their neck to create a double chin when they're beaming with happiness, and that their skin isn't made to be constantly tight and smooth, and that their legs are built to take them places, not to be looked at in disgust.

This world we live in is so incredible, but we are going to miss 90 per cent of it if we spend it focusing on our appearance instead of the happiness of ourselves and those around us.

You don't need to have a following to help create this change. If we all start showing

ourselves exactly as we are, then the change
will come. So who cares if the photo you want to
post isn't your best angle or you have a pimple
on your face? We're all real. We're all human.
Let's stop fooling each other into thinking we are
something else.

I STAND BY THAT message. Even now, years later, it speaks
to everything I'm passionate about. But I'd be lying if I said
I had it all figured out. The truth is I still have days when
I judge myself, days when I choose not to post a photo
that's captured an angle I don't like. A year after that shoot,
I was scrolling through old photos and found one shot I
had chosen not to share. I looked so incredibly happy in it
that, for a second, I wondered why I hadn't posted it — then
I remembered that, at the time, there had been a number of
things I didn't like about it, despite what I'd written in the
caption. I didn't like the way my stomach sat or the way my
chin was doubled or the way my hair was pulled back. It's
not that the other images I'd loved so much *didn't* show any
of these things, just that I'd decided I didn't like the angle of
this one particular image.

And you know what? A year on and I would have *killed*
to step back into that body, not just because of how fab
it looked but also because of how it moved. On the day I

rediscovered that image, I happened to be stuck in bed with a leg so swollen it wouldn't fit into my prosthetic. I couldn't have run along a sandy beach if I'd wanted to, and to realise that I hadn't liked a photo where I'd been so happy just because of the angle filled me with an overwhelming sense of sadness. Even while I'd been busy achieving something I'd only ever dreamt of, I'd still struggled to see anything other than aesthetic in that photo — and that broke my heart.

I don't want to write about how I have completely 'overcome my negative relationship with my body', because that just wouldn't be true. The reality is that it's a forever journey, a daily effort to find ways to not let the idea of what you should look like control you.

I share this story because I want you to know that none of us are perfect in any way. I'm definitely not, and that includes when it comes to loving myself all of the time. I don't want to write about how I have completely 'overcome my negative relationship with my body', because that just wouldn't be true. The reality is that it's a forever journey, a daily effort to find ways to not let the idea of what you should look like control you. I would hate for anyone to think that I just miraculously figured out how to live my life without making a single judgement of myself or ever comparing my life with others'. That's not realistic, so it shouldn't ever be the goal.

What I do believe is that none of those judgements or comparisons have to control your life. Now, whenever I do find myself having a judgemental thought, I turn it into a moment of appreciation for what I can do. So, *Your thigh is falling down and it looks weird in those jeans* becomes *Your thigh may be falling down, but you're able to stand and put one foot in front of the other.*

Try it. Instead of thinking negatively about how your body looks, maybe think of some things you're grateful that you can do. Try not to give that negative thought your time. Don't let it control your day. Because I can promise you that in a few years' time you won't miss a flat stomach as much as you'll miss the abilities you have now if they're ever lost.

THIS IS THE POINT where this sort of conversation can sometimes turn to the topics of 'self-love' and 'body positivity'. Both are concepts presented as ways to combat the illusion of 'perfect' that the online world projects. Self-love is pretty obvious — it's basically about showing yourself care — while body positivity is essentially a social movement advocating for wider representation of all kinds of bodies, regardless of size, shape, colour, gender or anything else. An idea behind both is that, instead of believing we must look a particular way and then beating ourselves up when we don't, we should turn the whole thing on its head and just love ourselves and our bodies. But, while I do believe that both self-love and body positivity are great messages, I also think they often get taken too far and too literally. I don't think it's realistic — or necessary — to love every single aspect of your body. That just places an insane amount of pressure on people because it asks them to go beyond simply living in their bodies. It's still focused totally on what your body looks like. Sitting in front of a mirror and forcing yourself to love the parts of your body you've been told not to love is still all about the exterior. And, as I've said, that's just not what's important.

For me and my body, self-love and body positivity just don't work. That's not to say that's true for anyone else — everyone has the right to find the messaging and way of being that works for them. But in my mind there's no getting around the fact that my body is incredibly unusual. I never find myself looking at my backwards foot in the mirror and thinking, *Damn, that's the most beautiful leg I've ever seen,* and I don't think I need to feel that way either. Instead, I look in the mirror and I think, *Yes, this leg is unusual and different, but it's the reason I am here. It's the reason I am able to walk around and live my life.* That, for me, is more than enough. The important thing isn't what my body looks like or even what it can do. What matters is how I live this life of mine in the body I have. What matters is simply *being* in my body.

No matter how honest someone promises to be online, they are still making choices about what they share and how they share it.

That's why I prefer to go with 'self-acceptance' and 'body neutrality'. I don't believe that, in order to stop loathing our bodies, we have to love every inch of them. My hope is that we can instead stop letting the way we look control everything. An incredible thing happens when you stop constantly trying to become the 'perfect' version of yourself and allow yourself to just be as you are in each moment.

I still believe we need to keep bringing our real selves to the online world if we want to cut through everything artificial, but I also think it's important to always remember that what's shown on social media is only ever going to be a small portion of someone's life. No matter how honest someone promises to be online, they are still making choices about what they share and how they share it. Those images from the Bondi shoot were all real and untouched — they showed my skin and my body and the way it moves, exactly as it is — but I still made a choice about which photos I would share with the world. I still chose not to share some because I didn't like them for superficial reasons.

It's all so complex — so, so complex. The relationships that many of us have with our bodies are, at least in part, a product of what the wider world has told us for too long. The negative things we think or do aren't directly our fault. We're acting, often subconsciously, on habits and mindsets and biases that have been passed down through generations. It's no wonder we are the way we are.

But it's our responsibility to break the chain, to ask ourselves the hard questions and force a different life for ourselves and for others.

At the end of the day, you live your life in this body of yours. Don't spend it at war.

TOWARDS THE END OF 2017, I got a message on Instagram from an account called Natural Model Management. I looked them up and saw they were an agency based in LA. The reason they'd got in touch, they said, was because they were interested in signing me. Did I want to chat?

It sounded too good to be true, and I knew that meant it quite possibly was. By this point, it wasn't unusual for me to get messages from people wanting me to sample their products or sell me a dream life, so I'd learnt to be a bit wary. But I'd always dreamt of living in LA, so I went and checked out the agency's Instagram profile, just to make sure. Everything looked pretty legitimate, so I agreed to jump on a video call with them.

And, turns out, it was real.

The two smiling faces that greeted me on the screen belonged to Katie Willcox, the founder of Natural Models, and Nikki Mann, the agency's head booker. I told them my story and explained how my hope, through my work, was to use my body to normalise being different. I even told them about my dream of changing the image on the billboard that the young girl in my mind kept walking past on her way to school, and mentioned in passing how I'd refused to wear shorts for eight years after losing my leg.

I must have said the right things because, before long, a contract came through to me. I was signed to Natural Models LA.

It was an exciting opportunity, to say the least, but there was still a bit of work to do before I'd be able to enjoy it fully. For starters, I needed to get a work visa sorted before I could go and live in the States, and that meant my modelling career there was going to be a slow build. But, while I waited for the paperwork to come through, I could still head over to LA to do some test shoots and start making plans with the Natural Models team for my future.

When I headed over to LA about six months after signing with them, I arrived to discover that Katie had already arranged a few photo shoots to help build up my modelling portfolio.

'And one of them is about wearing shorts,' she said. 'After you told me your story, I mentioned it to some of the other models and they all had their own stories about not wearing shorts.'

It was another pivotal moment for me. I realised that, even though my reason for covering up had been unique, I hadn't ever been alone in hiding part of my body from sight.

Their experiences and insecurities were all unique, she explained, and they were covering up for their own reasons, but the one thing we had in common was that we hadn't worn shorts for a huge portion of our lives. We'd each felt the need to hide our legs away, either out of fear of being judged or simply because we didn't feel good about our bodies. That had got Katie thinking that it'd be cool to do a shoot with all of us proudly wearing shorts. I was totally on board with the idea.

It was an incredible shoot to be part of, and for some of the models it was the first time in many years they'd shown their legs. It was another pivotal moment for me. I realised that, even though my reason for covering up had been unique, I hadn't ever been alone in hiding part of my body from sight. All of the other girls had two legs, but that didn't make any difference. They'd still felt so insecure about their legs they'd hidden them away.

My shorts story is a huge part of the bigger story I share. To me, it's an example of the fact that none of us are alone in having insecurities. I talk about it on Instagram often, and every time I do I'm flooded with messages from people who, to this day, don't wear shorts. Maybe they're trying to hide a scar or they feel their legs are too pale or too spotty. Perhaps they have cellulite or they don't like the way their legs have changed since giving birth. There are too many reasons to list, but they all lead to the same thing: people believing they shouldn't, or can't, wear shorts.

It's one more thing I want to change. We all have a right to wear shorts if we want to. So each summer, as the days get warmer and sunnier, I encourage everyone on Instagram to #wearthedamnshorts.

Life is far too short to hide away.

7

Jive
time

We humans are creatures of extremes. We only realise how strong we are when we have to be. We only learn how much we can truly handle when life puts us to the test. And we are all so much stronger than we give ourselves credit for.

I got to learn this at a really young age, and for that I consider myself pretty lucky.

I want to remind you that you are just as strong as I am. That you don't have to wait for adversity to hit in order to find that strength. It's already there within you.

Trust me.

Trust it.

WHEN I FIRST GOT my blade, it was because I wanted to run. I might not have been able to get it to carry me ten kilometres, but I did succeed in learning to do something with it that I'd thought I might never do again. And, little did I know, running wasn't the only ability my blade was going to grant me.

Early on in 2018, I went in for a meeting with my manager, Brooke, to talk about my plans and my work schedule for the coming year. Just before I was about to leave, he stopped me.

'One other thing,' he said. 'The producers of *Dancing with the Stars* have been in touch, and they want to know if you'd be interested in competing in it this year.'

'Am I being punked?' I said.

Brooke just shook his head. He was grinning.

'Um, okay,' I said, laughing. 'No thanks.'

I figured an offer to go on the New Zealand version of Britain's *Strictly Come Dancing* TV series was just another one of the outlandish opportunities I'd become accustomed to getting that never led to anything. I didn't really give it much thought.

But the next day I got a call from Brooke. 'The *Dancing with the Stars* producers really want to meet with you,' he said. 'They want to know if you'll do it or not.'

So it wasn't a joke.

While I'd stopped dancing after my rotationplasty, my little sister, Sophie-Rose, had gone on to become a professional dancer and had only recently stopped, so I actually knew a bit about the dancing world. But being on stage myself? No. When I lost my leg I also lost my ability to easily move quickly, let alone gracefully. I'd always been a bit envious of Soph's ability to move in the way she could. She is an amazing dancer.

'Brooke, you need to have a foot that allows you to pivot, a knee that bends, and an ankle that flexes and points if you want to dance at that level,' I said. 'My body just can't move like that.'

A small part of me really wanted to say yes — learning to dance would be an incredible challenge, the sort I'd usually jump at — but a bigger part of me was saying a firm no. I knew how difficult it would be to learn how to dance, and going through that process on live TV, bronzed and wearing Lycra, with the potential of falling on my face in front of millions of people? Not a chance. One day I'd learn to dance maybe, but not like that.

'Well, look,' Brooke replied, 'the meeting's set up anyway, so why don't you just go along and hear them out? It could always lead to other opportunities.'

'Okay,' I said, 'I'll go to the meeting. But on one condition: you have to understand I'm saying no to dancing.'

'Great!' said Brooke.

'So I'm not going to say yes,' I said.

'Sure thing,' said Brooke.

I could tell he was just playing along. It's almost like he'd sniffed the potential 'yes' that hovered behind my words. He knew me too well.

'This isn't like the other times,' I added, wanting to make things really clear. 'I'm not going to change my mind.'

'Of course not. See you at the meeting.'

THE MEETING WAS WITH the show's three producers. After we'd all shaken hands and sat down, they explained how the show worked and what would be involved. I smiled and nodded along, but I was only half listening — I'd already decided I wasn't going to do it, after all.

'And you'd get to dance for a charity of your choosing,' one of the producers said. I sat up a bit straighter. 'The money raised from viewers texting in to vote goes to the winners' chosen charities.'

That got my attention. *I could give back to the Child Cancer Foundation*, I thought, before reining in my emotions and reminding myself, *Jess, you can't dance with one leg.*

My brain went into overdrive then. It played out something like this:

You have to wear heels while ballroom dancing, and you can't wear high heels, remember?

And what if it's like running and your good leg can't cope? It's not worth the risk.

You can't even bend your knee properly. Wait, you don't even have a knee! Jess, do I need to remind you that you have a backwards foot for a knee and another foot made of plastic?!

You can't dance.

But maybe I can . . .

What! Why are you even starting to consider this?

It's fair to say that my brain can be a very busy place. It's also fair to say that nine times out of ten I ignore a lot of what it tells me.

I soon realised that the only reason I was saying no was because I believed I couldn't dance. I was afraid of failing, afraid that my leg would hold me back. That was the moment I knew I was going to say yes: the second that one part of my mind starts to say I can't do something, another part is already rising to the challenge of proving that part wrong.

I have to show myself I can do that thing, or at least give it a determined try.

What's the worst that could happen? I asked myself. *Sure, you could fall flat on your face on national TV, but hey! You faced cancer! You know it could always be worse.*

I'm apparently unable to settle for the simple life — and Brooke knew this. Over our years working together, this exact same sequence has played out more times than I can count: he presents me with an opportunity, I freak out and say no, he convinces me to do it and I eventually agree, then I come to tell him afterwards that it's the best thing I've ever done and I want to do it all over again.

'Okay,' I said to the producers. 'I'll give it a go.'

'Fantastic!' They were all beaming.

> **This exact same sequence has played out more times than I can count: Brooke presents me with an opportunity, I freak out and say no, he convinces me to do it and I eventually agree, then I come to tell him afterwards that it's the best thing I've ever done and I want to do it all over again.**

'But, before we make it official,' I said, 'I need to make sure I am actually physically capable of dancing.'

'Of course,' one of them replied. 'We can arrange for you

to do a private session with a dance teacher in the next few days to see how you get on. How does that sound?'

'That works,' I replied. 'And so long as I can do the basic steps, I'll go on the show. Count me in.'

When I got back to my car, I opened our family chat. 'Life just got weirder,' I wrote. 'I am going to be on *Dancing with the Stars*.'

Almost immediately, replies popped up on the screen from my sisters. They'd both sent me gifs of ballroom dancers falling to the floor mid-routine. Gotta love sisters.

MY PRIVATE DANCE SESSION went ahead without a hitch. An incredible woman who was to be the head dancer in charge of choreography for the show took me through some basic steps, and they were all really achievable. I wore my everyday prosthetic because I felt I needed a solid foundation to be able to move, and it was fine. Knowing how unstable my blade was, I considered dancing on it for only a moment before dismissing the idea.

And, just like that, my next adventure kicked off. All of a sudden, I was busy going to photo shoots and filming TV commercials in the lead-up to the official announcements of that season's dancers. I still remember the day I met my dance partner, Jonny Williams. I was a bit nervous. What if we didn't get on? This was someone I was going to have to spend a lot of time with, day in, day out, and in my most vulnerable state. With cameras following my every step, I walked into the dance studio and introduced myself to him.

'I see you brought a spare leg,' he said with a smirk, gesturing to my blade, which was tucked under my arm. Even though I knew it was unlikely that I'd be dancing in the blade, I'd taken it just in case. I'd never done this dancing thing before, after all. And when Jonny made that remark about my leg, any worries I'd had about my dance partner vanished. I knew we were going to get along just fine.

Jonny was by far the most experienced dancer on the show, and we had four weeks of pre-training together before the live shows started. That's four weeks in which to go from having never danced with my prosthetic to dancing live on national TV.

When Jonny made that remark about my leg, any worries I'd had about my dance partner vanished. I knew we were going to get along just fine.

It's probably a good thing the training was so demanding, as I don't think the enormity of what I was embarking on really hit me. (Honestly, that period in my life was such a whirlwind that I *still* don't think it has hit me.) Right from day one, we didn't take a single day off. To begin with, we trained for four hours a day, but within a week that had climbed to six hours. Pretty soon, we were doing a steady ten to fourteen hours a day.

If you've never watched *Dancing with the Stars* (no judgement — I hadn't either before I went on the show), the way it works is that celebrities are paired with professional dancers and must perform a dance of a particular style each week to both a panel of judges and, you know, the nation. Viewers vote by text on who they think should make it through to the following week, and the couple with the combined lowest score from the public and the judges at the end of each episode is eliminated. As the producers had mentioned in my meeting with them, proceeds from the phone voting go towards each celebrity's charity of choice, so there's an extra incentive to last as long as you can in the competition — the longer you go without getting voted off, the more money you make for your charity.

For week one, the style of dance that Jonny had chosen for us was the rumba. It's a softer style of rhythmic dance, and we had three weeks to work on it — by far the longest we'd get for any dance in the entire season. Once the show started, we could only really work a week or so out, because we never knew whether we'd make it through to the following week.

For those first three weeks learning the rumba with Jonny, I wore my everyday prosthetic. I struggled to move gracefully on it, given that my prosthetic foot doesn't offer any kind of flexion, but every time I wondered whether I should give the blade a go, I talked myself out of it. I was sure its instability would cause even more issues than my everyday prosthetic. I felt stuck between a rock and a hard place, but I persevered.

To add to that, I had to wear ballet slippers instead of high heels. I'd never been able to wear heels due to my prosthetic's lack of ankle mobility, and it was something that had driven me mad. Dancing was no different. I hated wearing those little slippers. I felt so ungraceful.

All of a sudden, my running leg had transformed into a dancing leg. All I had to do now was to actually try dancing in it.

Just six days out from our first live performance, I finally managed to get the routine down. That day, something came over me.

'Let's give it a go with my blade,' I said to Jonny.

I had a feeling it probably wasn't going to go well, but I just needed to try so I could stop wondering. I put my blade on, then grabbed a dancing high heel that was lying around the studio. And do you know what? As soon as I'd squished my foot into the heel and stood up, I discovered it was at the perfect height to level out my hips and legs. All of a sudden, my running leg had transformed into a dancing leg.

All I had to do now was to actually try dancing in it.

During our first run-through with the blade, I was a little shaky. It was just like I was nine again and learning to walk after my surgery. I felt a bit like a giraffe on ice, but we gave it a few more tries. That was all it took for both me and Jonny to realise we were heading in the right direction.

'I think I can just change legs depending on the style of dance each week,' I said to him. 'But let's go with the blade for the rumba.'

'Okay, let's do it,' he agreed.

I so clearly remember those final days before our first dance. We had less than a week left, and learning the dance on a different leg meant basically starting from scratch. At the same time, I also had to learn how to walk in a high heel. At the age of 25, it was something I'd never done before. Luckily, Jonny was well used to teaching young dancers how to walk in heels, and he soon had me doing laps of the studio, perfecting my prance. Every session that week caused my high-heeled left foot to go numb, but aside from that I actually felt really comfortable in my new shoe. I think my many, many years of adjusting to a new way of moving served me well when it came to adapting to the high heel. It was such an improvement on the ballet slipper, and I felt so much more graceful.

For the rumba, our finishing move involved me doing a

kind of spin where I ended half crouched on Jonny's knee, leaning fully to one side, while he held my waist (I promise it was more elegant than it sounds). In the days leading up to our performance, we practised this move over and over and over again, until I felt like I knew it inside out. Then, just four days out, disaster struck. I suddenly began to suffer excruciating pain in my ribs — I think that hitting them over and over again during the spin had simply become too much. I somehow managed to carry on until the day before our TV performance, when we did a run-through at the studio where the live show would be filmed. During the dance, my diaphragm went into a spasm, so on the morning of our first-ever live show I found myself sitting in A & E at the hospital, being prescribed pain meds for a broken rib. I headed straight to the studio afterwards, and spent the rest of the day in full hair and make-up, with an ice pack attached to my rib. I was so nervous that this was going to affect our performance.

Then, finally, the moment was upon us. It was time to dance.

I had thought I was prepared. I felt like I could do the dance with my eyes closed. Jonny and I had rehearsed it on the dance floor, and I had imagined the live audience being there. I was starting to get used to the six cameras that followed my every move. I knew where the judges would be sitting. I was familiar with the lights, the glitter, the Lycra, the make-up. I was used to the way my blade's rubber sole stuck to the dance floor and to having almost no feeling in either of my feet. I trusted Jonny more than anything.

But nothing can prepare you for the moment you step out onto a dance floor to the cheers and whistles of an overexcited audience that includes your proud parents. You take your position. You can feel the blood pumping through your body. For a split second you wonder how you're going to get through, you wonder how you got here, and you realise there's no turning back now. The floor manager counts you down before the cameras start feeding to the live TV, and at the same time the music starts. And then you start dancing.

But nothing can prepare you for the moment you step out onto a dance floor to the cheers and whistles of an overexcited audience that includes your proud parents.

I twirled around the dance floor, a high heel on one foot and a blade on the other, landing every single move, including our final spin. The whole thing was over as suddenly as it had begun.

Four weeks of hard work for one and a half minutes.

Later, I saw a photo of Jonny and me in our final position. I am beaming from ear to ear, looking directly at the judges.

We had done it.

BY THE TIME I got home that night, Mum and Dad had the whole thing ready for me to watch. They'd recorded it and had already watched it again themselves, several times over.

It was only then, seeing myself live on TV, that I realised exactly what I'd just achieved. I had danced, on my blade, on live TV, in front of millions of people. I know that might sound a bit dramatic — it's just a TV show after all — but it really was so much more than that to me. It was as if every moment of doubt, every minute I'd spent on the sidelines and every time I'd persevered had all led to this.

And, after the remaining competitors for that week had danced the following night, Jonny and I discovered we'd topped the leader board. That was when things really got real. The show became my life, and my weekly schedule looked something like this:

Tuesday to Friday: practising our dance routine at Jonny's studio.

Saturday: rehearsing at the performance studio and getting my all-important weekly spray tan.

Sunday: somewhere between twelve and fourteen hours in the studio leading up to that night's live show.

Monday: the elimination show.

Then, if we made it through to the next week, we'd be back at it on Tuesday, ready to learn a new dance by Friday, no matter how exhausted we were. The whole time, I never really knew when it would all come to an end. Each week presented a new challenge, as Jonny picked a new style of dance from the list for us to explore, but week after week we somehow nailed it.

> **It's my mission to show people that we're all different, that we can all give anything we dream of our best shot, even if that means doing it our own way.**

I almost forgot a world existed outside of the show — never before had I felt so in my element. Here I was doing something, yet again, that I had once thought I could never do. It's my mission to show people that we're all different, that we can all give anything we dream of our best shot, even if that means doing it our own way, and the show was helping me do just that. Every week I encountered fans of all ages — everyone from my grandparents' friends to three-year-olds I'd never met before — who said they were inspired by what I was doing. It meant so much to have kids giving me the drawings they'd done of me dancing with my blade. It was incredible to know that I was showing young people someone who looked different to what they were used to seeing on mainstream TV.

When I'd first agreed to do the show, the thing I'd been most concerned about was my good leg. I was nervous that my calf, which had only just fully healed from the stress fracture, would give out just like it had with running. But I needn't have worried — my left leg was incredible. I had regular chiropractor appointments to help me manage the tension in it, and each week I was pleasantly surprised by how well it was coping given the load it was suddenly taking. Most people with two legs wouldn't be able to push their body to that extreme for up to fourteen hours a day for three solid months, yet I was somehow managing to do it mostly on one leg. It's amazing how the body can adapt, especially when adrenaline is involved. Even so, I don't think you can take on a whole new sport in such a short space of time and get away without a mark — I admit that I did end up losing all sensation in the big toe on my high-heeled foot for the entire season and a few months after *Dancing with the Stars* finished, but I pushed on.

Somehow, Jonny and I made it all the way to week nine, the second-to-last episode of the season. How we made it that far was beyond me, but there we were. On this particular week we didn't get to choose our dance style and were assigned the jive — the style I'd been avoiding all season, in the hope I wouldn't have to do it at all. To me, a jive is basically a lot of up-and-down running and bouncing movements, where you bring your knees almost up to your chest and you're somehow supposed to make it all look coordinated.

Jonny and I had given it a go early on in the show and had discovered that it was the one style that probably wasn't going to end well for me. At first I'd thought maybe it wouldn't be so bad, given I had a spring for a foot, but it turned out that I had very little control over the direction my blade would bounce me in. That made doing a jive way more difficult than any of the other styles, and I honestly didn't see how it would even be physically possible for me.

So, when I learnt we were doing a jive for week nine, I admit I did think about giving up for a second.

**Things looked nearly impossible.
But if there's one thing I'd got
exceptionally good at by that point, it
was surviving the nearly impossible.**

Then we discovered that week's dance was also to be themed 'Most Memorable Year'. We'd known a themed week was coming at some point, and we'd planned on doing a slow, soft dance about 2001, the year my life changed. Well, there's no way you can softly dance a jive.

Things looked nearly impossible.

But if there's one thing I'd got exceptionally good at by that point, it was surviving the nearly impossible.

LET'S REWIND FOR A minute, all the way back to Monday, 23 July 2001, when I was just eight years old, four months after I'd stood on that soccer ball and broken my femur and eleven days after I'd been diagnosed with cancer. That Monday, my family and I celebrated my big sister Abby's eleventh birthday. We had a party at home, with cake and friends. My parents were doing their best to keep everything normal, despite the fact that our lives had just become anything but.

The next day, I was admitted to Ward 27B at Starship Hospital in the inner Auckland suburb of Grafton. Over the next nine months, this place would become more familiar to me than my own home, and I soon had my room at the hospital set up as though it was: my duvet, my favourite fluffy pink star pillow, my growing collection of teddy bears, Bunny. The only thing that was different from home was that I had a TV in my room, a McDonald's downstairs and a nurse's bell attached to my bed. Oh, and I was also there to begin nine harrowing months of chemotherapy.

At eight, I was completely oblivious to how hard life in general can be, let alone how hard my own life was about to get. My parents, however, would have had more of an idea. Ever since the meeting with the oncologist just a few weeks earlier, when they'd learnt their little girl had cancer and was most likely going to lose her leg, their view of the difficult road ahead would have become increasingly clear.

In that meeting, the oncologist had explained my prognosis. When I asked Dad about this recently, he said that he and Mum were told the survival rate of osteosarcoma was pretty low and fluky at the time, but that doctors were getting better at managing both the cancer itself and the effects of the chemo they used to treat it. Since osteosarcoma is a bone cancer, Dad said, my doctors were very worried about it spreading and getting into other parts of my system, as that would have just made the outlook even worse. So their plan was to use chemo to attack and reduce the cancer, both before and after amputating my leg. They felt this would give me the best chance of survival.

'The "cool" thing about having cancer in an extremity,' Dad said, 'is that the extremity can be removed, and that removes all issues if the cancer hasn't spread elsewhere.'

The 'extremity' in this case was, of course, my leg.

After explaining this pretty grim prognosis, the oncologist then outlined my treatment plan. He spelt out what we should expect from the chemo and how our lives were going to look. My medical notes from that appointment include a long list of the side effects he told my parents about — such things as bone marrow depression, mouth sores ('occasionally severe'), nausea, vomiting, diarrhoea, skin rashes, decreased liver function, brain damage, liver damage, kidney damage and hair loss.

There's nothing gentle or caring about cancer. This was

our new, harsh reality: the reality of childhood cancer.

It must have been around this time, when my parents realised just how many horrible treatments I was about to undergo, that Mum decided it might be a good idea to give me something to aim for at the end of it all.

'You can pick anything you like,' she said to me. 'Anything at all.'

I thought about it for a moment, then said decisively, 'Rainbow's End. I want to go to Rainbow's End.'

Mum decided it might be a good idea to give me something to aim for at the end of it all. 'You can pick anything you like,' she said.

Look, I was eight. A trip to Auckland's main theme park was about the biggest, coolest thing I could think of right then.

'Think bigger,' Mum said. 'What's something that you really, really want? Something that you've always dreamt of?'

I thought a bit harder this time, and then I said, 'A dog!'

So it was decided: once I'd finished the chemo and got out of hospital, however long that took, I would get a dog. For every treatment I had to endure, Mum would bring along a dog book to distract me, and we'd flick through looking at all the different breeds. Almost immediately, I got my heart set on a golden retriever, but such a massive dog would have been comically inappropriate for a newly one-legged nine-year-old, so Mum gently suggested I pick something a bit smaller. I eventually settled on a Cavalier King Charles spaniel. I had to wait for a long time and go through a lot before I got my puppy, but the day finally came just before I went back to school in 2002. I called him Charlie, and the two of us pretty much grew up together and did everything together, including learning to walk at the same time. He was a huge part of my life. (And, actually, he passed away only just before I started *Dancing with the Stars*. Losing him was truly one of the hardest things I'd been through at that point.)

But back to chemo. The very first procedure I had to go through before my treatment could start was to have a port-a-cath inserted just beneath the skin on my chest. I still remember the doctor showing the port to me. It was a little plastic circle about the size of a 50-cent coin and 1.5 centimetres high. There was a thin, flexible cord coming off to one side, and a small gel-like pad in the middle. A port-a-cath is basically a small device that means your doctors just have to prick and prod you in one spot — necessary when it comes to something like chemo, as so many drugs have to be injected that your veins would be ruined otherwise. The round plastic bit — the port — sits just under the skin on the right side of your chest, and the cord — the catheter — is then threaded into the large vein above the right side of your heart, called the vena cava. It can stay there for years if needed, and makes it much easier to both inject medications and also draw blood.

The surgery to insert the port-a-cath was minor, and by that time I'd already had enough surgeries that I didn't think too much of it anyway. For me, the scariest part of the whole thing was the first time a needle was inserted into my port, ahead of my first chemo session. A nurse numbed the spot where the port pushed my skin out into a visible lump, then inserted the needle. It hurt a bit, but it was over quickly, a bit like getting a piercing. The nurse then secured the needle in place with a clear, sterile plaster — I've had so many of these plasters applied that I can still smell them today. The needle was attached to an intravenous (IV) line that would, the following day, be hooked up to a chemotherapy bag hanging from a pole. I would lie in bed while the drugs were pumped along that line, straight into my little body.

My chemo schedule chopped and changed a bit, depending on how my body was handling the treatment, but essentially I would go into the hospital every other week and spend a whole week there receiving chemotherapy. Before each round of chemo, I had to have a needle inserted into my port. Then I spent the in-between weeks at home. As the months accrued, so did the promised side effects: the vomiting, the nausea, the mouth ulcers, the diarrhoea, the loss of appetite, the fever, the chills, the fatigue, the weight loss, the hair loss. When I first read in my medical notes that losing my leg had actually been on the cards from day one, I wondered why my doctors hadn't just gone ahead and amputated it straight away to save me all the pain of chemotherapy. Chemo is the worst. I'm sure you know that. It doesn't discern between what kinds of cells it attacks — so, while it's trying to kill off the bad cells, it's also busy attacking all the good cells in your body. Often the side effects of chemo make you feel sicker than the cancer itself does. But, of course, my doctors had to at least try to shrink the cancer before they took my leg, and they also couldn't take the risk that it wasn't already invading other areas of my young body.

As the months accrued, so did the promised side effects: the vomiting, the nausea, the mouth ulcers, the diarrhoea, the loss of appetite, the fever, the chills, the fatigue, the weight loss, the hair loss.

On Ward 27B, it was easy to tell who the new patients were, because they still had their hair. Even as I began to rack up one side effect after another, and even though I saw a constant stream of children also going through chemo and losing their hair, I still wondered if I might dodge that particular bullet. Surely it wouldn't happen to me. Surely

I wouldn't have to be one of those kids who tosses up between a wig and a bandana. Then one day I woke up and found a clump of hair on my pillow. The next day, more hair came away in my hands while Mum was helping me shower. Each day it got worse, until eventually I looked like I'd had a run-in with a bad hairdresser wielding a pair of hedge clippers. Soon it was all gone — including my eyebrows, my eyelashes and every single other hair that had tried to grow on my body. My family and some of our closest friends made a big effort to turn it into a sort of special occasion, bringing treats and bandanas. Thanks to their love and support, I don't remember being horrifically upset about finally losing all my hair.

Part of me began to forget what life before cancer had been like. I forgot that there was a life outside the hospital and the treatments and the side effects.

It also probably helped that none of my new hospital friends had any hair either. While I still missed school and my old friends, those things soon started to fade in my mind. Part of me began to forget what life before cancer had been like. I forgot that there was a life outside the hospital and the treatments and the side effects. For me, there were no more morning-tea or lunch breaks, no more playing outside. My days were mostly spent in a hospital bed instead of a classroom chair, and the hospital hallways became my playground whenever I had enough energy to get up. Some days I went to the classroom on the other side of the ward to paint a picture or read. My new friends were all attached to IV drips, just like me, and they were all battling some kind of illness. Some of them wore bandanas, others bore big scars, and others had their bodies encased in plaster.

One day, a friend called Hannah and I spent time coming up with acrostics to remember our National Health Index numbers, which were on the patient ID bands we wore around our wrists. I can't remember mine exactly, but I think it went something like 'Goat Donkey Unicorn' followed by a series of numbers. It certainly wasn't the way I had passed my time at school, and Hannah — who was having treatment for a brain tumour — was going through something every bit as difficult as I was. But we were still just little kids. We still managed to find ways to have fun.

I remember a nurse coming in to check on me one day. She pulled her lanyard out of her pocket, and alongside her swipe key I saw she had about ten different key rings hanging there.

'What are all those for?' I asked. 'They look really heavy.' It seemed like a ridiculous weight to carry around in your pocket.

'I use them to help kids take their minds off the different procedures they have to get done,' she explained. 'Would you like to have a look?'

'Yes, please,' I said, then inspected each key ring closely. I thought they were pretty cool. 'Thanks,' I said, passing them back to her. Then I added, 'I bet I can collect even more than you have!'

I was clearly missing the competitive aspect of playing sport.

She smiled. 'Game on!'

And so began my key-ring mission. Word got around, and soon any time anyone came to visit they would bring me a key ring. Dad's work colleagues gave them to him to pass on to me. I started to get packages in the post from family friends, and inside I'd find a Mickey Mouse key ring along with a letter telling me all about their vacation to Disneyland. It wasn't long before I had a bunch of key rings from all over the world. We hung them off the pole holding my chemo bag, and by the time my treatment had finished they draped down onto the floor. Mum and I counted them, and all up I'd managed to collect over 300 key rings. I well and truly won that bet!

When I was in the hospital, my parents would take turns sleeping there with me while the other stayed at home with Abby and Sophie-Rose. Everything was topsy-turvy for everyone. They had to work out how to juggle caring for two kids at home with caring for one in hospital, and Dad also still had to go to work. Almost straight away, Nana moved up from Wellington to live with us so that Abby and Soph would always have someone at home with them if our parents couldn't be there. Nana was also often the one who would come running to me when I was at home and the side effects got too much. Grandma, Dad's mum, was also always around. She'd swing by the house to drop off mac and cheese (our favourite), and she'd come in to spend time with me at the hospital so that Mum and Dad could go and do all the other things they still needed to do.

While I'm sure it was nice for Mum and Dad to have me at home and be able to sleep in their own bed in between my chemo sessions, it was also scary. At the hospital, we were surrounded 24/7 by professionals who knew how to manage my symptoms. At home we had none of that. It was just my parents and Nana. The chemo had blitzed my immune system, so there was a really high risk of me getting an infection if I was exposed to bacteria. Everything had to be cleaned hourly. I still remember Mum and Nana scrubbing every surface and door handle whenever they entered or left a room. To add to that, I had to be watched constantly, given all sorts of pills, and repeatedly taken to the bathroom to vomit. Throughout the night, my various symptoms would wake me up hourly. To begin with, I slept alone in my room, which was near Abby's but at the opposite end from Mum and Dad's. The house wasn't big, but my parents were far enough away that they'd only hear me in the night if (a) I was screaming and (b) they were already awake. It was easier for me to just wake my big sister and send her down to get someone, but that wasn't ideal for an eleven-year-old with school the next day. So Dad ended up sleeping in my room most nights.

I have no idea how Mum has dealt with it for so long, but my dad is a seriously heavy snorer. Sometimes I didn't wake him up for help but just to get him to stop snoring. I soon developed a simple but highly effective trick, which I called the Teddy-bear System, that consisted of chucking Bunny at Dad. I used this trick at home and at the hospital. Bunny was soft, except for his paws, which were filled with lots of little beans. I'm sure it wasn't very comfortable to get whacked with them in the middle of the night, but it wasn't very comfortable listening to Dad snore either! I still remember lying there in the middle of the night, holding Bunny in a position ready to throw, waiting and hoping that the sickness would pass or that Dad's snoring would end. I always felt bad for disturbing his sleep, so I'd wait until I really, really needed him before I smacked him in the head with a flying toy.

Life wasn't just different for me. It was different for my whole family. That's the thing about cancer: it's not biased. It wreaks havoc in the lives of every single person who comes near it. Only one person might be physically fighting the disease, but everyone around them is fighting too — just in a different way. Everyone feels the effects.

I SOMETIMES FEEL LIKE I've lived a lot of my life in hindsight. By the time I turned nine, I had faced more adversity than some people do in their whole lives. I just wouldn't learn the full implications of everything I'd been through until long after it had all happened.

> **Before I'd even had the chance to dream, I'd already learnt to sidestep obstacles and take detours. I found out how hard life can get before I knew just how good it can be, and that changed my perspective on everything.**

We all have dreams of what we hope our lives will look like, but sometimes the images in our heads don't match our realities. Life places obstacles in front of us that we never expect or plan for. We manage to jump over some, but others send us in a new direction completely. When I was told I had cancer, I was too young to dream. I mean, I had dreams, but not real ones — not dreams of what my future could look like. I was only eight. So, before I'd even had the chance to dream, I'd already learnt to sidestep obstacles and take detours. I found out how hard life can get before I knew just how good it can be, and that changed my perspective on everything.

As I write about my cancer journey now, I can't help wondering how I would have felt if I'd had to go through it when I was older. I wouldn't have been so naive. I would have properly understood everything. I would have known how things might end. I would have been much more afraid. It's a bit like being in an aeroplane, actually. As an adult, I have a pretty strong fear of flying, but when I was a kid I never worried about the what ifs or the maybes. I just went along with the ride — being on a plane was just one big, exciting experience. Even turbulence was fun — it felt like a roller coaster. Then I got older, and suddenly being on a plane was petrifying. As soon as turbulence hits now, I'm terrified that the plane is going to go down. From the outside, nothing about the experience has changed. It's exactly the same. The only thing that's different is me.

Adults seem to be obsessed with going through pain and hardship twice — once when we fear a thing happening, and again if it actually happens. When children are naive, it's because they haven't learnt enough to fear the world. That's the beauty of children, and it's the beauty of naivety. Little Jess's naivety is the reason I'm still standing today. To be honest, the process of writing this all down has been much harder than going through my memories. My medical notes have given me a clearer sense of hindsight. I've had to feel it all again. It's hard to relive it, but I'll be forever grateful that I never had to understand it all until much later.

Every now and again, I look through photos from that time and begin to reminisce. I find comfort in doing this. It's a gentle reminder that gives me a deep sense of just how strong that little kid was. And it also reminds me just how strong I am now.

I don't think of the year 2001 as a sad and sombre time in my life. No, I think of it as the moment when I realised what I was capable of. I see it as a chapter in my story. It's the year I showed cancer who's boss. It's the year I managed to get back up. If I could get through all that, then I can get through anything.

You can too.

WHEN JONNY AND I learnt that we were going to have to do a jive for week nine of *Dancing with the Stars* and that it would have to be themed 'Most Memorable Year', we had to work out what we were going to do pretty quickly.

But how do you capture everything I went through in 2001 in a bouncy, upbeat dance number? And was I even going to be able to pull it off physically?

One thing I did know: it was going to be hard. But by this point challenges had become my thing. I quickly let go of the idea of doing a sad, sombre dance, and I reminded myself that 2001 was the year that I survived, the year that I learnt just how strong I am. And that's what I needed to show in our dance. From there, it all started to fall into place. We picked Elton John's 'I'm Still Standing' as our track. (It was either that or 'Footloose', but we weren't sure people would get the reference.) Then we got started on the choreography.

The first day of dancing the jive was rough. Time and time again, I wondered how it was all going to come together in just four days, but I stuck at it. Somehow, I managed to figure out how to use the blade in the way the dance required, then Jonny and I adapted the moves we needed. Every night that week was a late one. Everything would start to come together to a certain point, and then it would fall apart and I would start doubting myself all over again.

This dance meant so much — the meaning behind it, the fact that we had made it so far in the competition, the pressure of wanting to get through to the final — but we were both exhausted after three months of non-stop dancing. The night before the final rehearsal, I honestly wondered whether this mountain might be one I wouldn't scale. I couldn't seem to get my legs to move in the way I wanted them to, but that was too bad. We didn't have any more time left to work on it. We had done the best we could, and that's all we could do. I was happy with that. Even if the worst happened and I got out on the dance floor and fell flat on my face, I would know I'd given it my all (and I could at least hope for some sympathy votes).

When show day dawned, I was more nervous than I'd ever been before.

I could barely believe it. I'd just danced the jive. I'll remember that feeling for the rest of my life.

I remember walking out onto the dance floor, and the applause dying down gradually until the room was stone quiet. I took my position in front of the judges, while Jonny took his on the other side of the dance floor. This was the first time we hadn't started a dance together, and that just made everything so much worse. I was so worried that the music would start and, without having Jonny there to guide me, I'd miss the first beat.

Then the lights came on.

The music belted.

Right on cue, I took my first few short steps towards Jonny, and we started dancing.

The audience cheered.

One minute and 30 seconds later, it was all over.

I could barely believe it. I'd just danced the jive.

I'll remember that feeling for the rest of my life.

We got our first 10 that night. We were also told it was one of the best jives of the season, and we found ourselves through to finals week. In the end, we placed third overall.

Third!

And to think I had started out wondering whether I'd even be able to dance.

I HOLD SO MUCH joy for that time in my life. I genuinely wish I could do it all over again. For a while I wondered why. It was just a TV show, after all — but then I realised that it wasn't *just* a TV show for me. In fact, it had nothing at all to do with being on TV and everything to do with making it through three months of tough physical challenges and surprising myself with just what I was capable of. I was training like an athlete. I was putting my body to the test. I was doing something that I'd never thought I would be able to do. And, a few months after the show had finished, we learnt that we had raised $55,000 for the Child Cancer Foundation. It took months afterwards for me to believe what I'd achieved, and even now I still have to sit and pause, and reflect on just how incredible it all was.

But I'm not actually here to brag about all of the things I've been able to do. This isn't really about me. It's about all of us. I want my life and my adversity to be an example. I got dealt a really average hand and I've had to navigate some tough paths to get here, but I would do it all over again. I truly believe that the mountains placed in my way were put there so that I can show others it's possible to climb their own. I am not what happened to me, but I am the person who is still standing through it all.

Whenever I hear people say you shouldn't be defined by your adversity, I just think, *Of course you're going to be defined by it.* It's a part of your life, a piece of the puzzle that makes up your story. The key is that you get to choose the definition. You have the pen in your hand. You dictate how that story turns out, regardless of what you went through. This is a conversation I have with myself often. My whole life has been about my leg, to the point where, if someone asks about my life, I struggle not to say 'I lost my leg to cancer when I was a kid' in the first sentence. But, at the end of the day, that's because that is the biggest part of my story. Sure, I am so much more than just a girl who lost her leg, but my god, is that a huge part of me. It's where all of my most profound lessons have come from. It's how I became the person I am today.

It's okay to look back on what you went through and write the narrative in your own words. So what if it's different from how others would write it? If you've been through something you didn't think you could survive, welcome to the human experience. The challenges are there to show you who you are, to show you what you are made of.

And between all of the difficult moments, don't forget to live a life. Bake brownies on a Sunday morning just because you feel like it. Laugh uncontrollably at something silly. Take a walk. Look at the trees. Hug your family. Find someone that feels like love. Read a book. Just live. Don't allow your brain to keep you trapped in a hardship that has passed. Hate it, scream at it, get mad, but please, do not forget to live.

8

Making a stand

Honestly, modelling is scary. Nine times out of ten I'm completely out of my comfort zone. I have to fight through tokenism a lot. I show even more of myself than I ever thought I would. But I have a purpose and a mission.

I want everyone, young and old, to see different bodies everywhere — in the media, in magazines, in advertising, on billboards. We have been fed a lie that 'different' isn't completely normal, and I want to change that. I want to normalise different.

There is no 'standard' of beauty. There is no right or wrong way to have a body. The way we look is of so little importance it shouldn't even matter. I look different from the majority of the population, but *newsflash* so do you. So does the person next to you. So does the next person.

Celebrate your difference. Don't let society make you think you need to be anything other than what you are. Don't waste your life being focused only on how you look.

You're so much more than that.

BY THE TIME *Dancing with the Stars* finished, I was still waiting for my visa to live and work in LA. Luckily, I was more than busy enough with everything I was doing here at home.

Just a week after the show wrapped, a women's lifestyle magazine got in touch about doing a write-up on my story and what I'd achieved. There was a photo shoot to go alongside the feature, and I remember turning up and feeling incredible, both physically and mentally. I wore my blade, as the shoot was sports-based, and most of the clothing I wore was workout leggings and crop tops. A month or so later, the images came out in the magazine and I felt beyond proud. I emailed the company to request the photos for my modelling portfolio, and a day or so later they sent them through. There were two folders attached to the email I received. One contained the images I'd seen in the magazine, while the other was called 'unworked on images'. *What are those ones?* I wondered as I clicked on the folder to open it. What I saw were the same images from the magazine, but with a slight but significant difference: these ones looked much more like me.

That was when I realised that the images I'd seen in the magazine had been photoshopped. You might be wondering why I hadn't noticed this as soon as I'd looked at them, but the changes were minor — I had fewer moles, my waist and legs had been slimmed, and my skin was smooth and glowing. In fact, in the past I've seen unretouched photos and found myself thinking, *Wow, I have more moles than I realised* or *Oh, I'm curvier there than I thought.* The truth is we very rarely see ourselves from all angles in the way that we can in photos.

I felt really frustrated that images of my body had been changed without my permission. It was a weird feeling, thinking that someone else had wielded a 'magic wand' to remove what they perceived as my imperfections. I felt like someone was pointing out the things that were wrong with my body, and they were all things that I'd never even known were a problem. What really hurt was realising that someone felt they could tell me the right way to live in this body of mine. What hurt even more was knowing the number of people who would have seen those images and believed that's what I really looked like. Here I was, telling my story, being raw in a photo shoot, showing my leg — an insecurity I'd held for so many years — and that still wasn't good enough.

It was the subtleness of the changes that most got to me. Even I, the person who lived in this body, had been fooled by them. I'd believed the way I looked was just a matter of some good lighting and a bit of make-up. That's the problem with a lot of image retouching: it's so subtle that we don't even notice it. It tricks us into thinking that things like moles, pores, hair and wrinkles aren't as common as they are. We might be able to see straight through overly photoshopped images, but we have no idea just how many of the images we see every day have been retouched. These subtly retouched images make us believe that kind of perfection is achievable when it's not. The model doesn't even look that perfect in reality.

At first, I didn't know what to do. I'd just assumed my images wouldn't be retouched without my permission, and I wasn't especially mad at the company or the photographer — I understood that they were working in a world where perfected images were the norm.

Maybe I should have spoken up ahead of the photo shoot? I thought. *Maybe I was meant to say that I didn't want my images photoshopped?*

I momentarily thought about just leaving it, writing it off as a lesson to make my expectations clearer in future.

But then I felt a huge sense of responsibility. Every day I was busy talking about how our world needed to show more diversity, how we needed to be more 'real' on social media, and how we needed to normalise imperfections and differences. How could I let people see a version of myself that didn't physically exist? It felt wrong. It felt hypocritical of me not to speak up. Given the magazine had already gone to print, I knew I couldn't retract those particular images, but I hoped that maybe I could use them as an example of why we needed to change things.

Every day I was busy talking about how our world needed to show more diversity, how we needed to be more 'real' on social media, and how we needed to normalise imperfections and differences. How could I let people see a version of myself that didn't physically exist? It felt wrong. It felt hypocritical of me not to speak up.

I thought of that young girl walking past that billboard in my mind, and I was unsettled beyond belief. Finally, we were starting to see some changes in the industry, with curve models and different ethnicities getting better representation, but what was the point if they were still being photoshopped so they just represented another 'ideal'?

It felt like saying, 'Here, we're ticking the box to make you happy and give you representation, but we are still going to make it unattainable and unrealistic.' I just couldn't sit there and do nothing. I knew I needed to use this experience to demand change.

First, I went to the publishing company. I asked why the images had been retouched and explained that I wasn't happy about it. They told me it was just part of the process. I sat on this for a while, wanting to speak up but unsure how to go about it.

I also mentioned it to Brooke, and one morning he gave me a call to say he'd been talking to a reporter he knew who wanted to do a piece on it. I was reluctant at first, but Brooke encouraged me to share my side of the story, so I agreed as long as I didn't have to name the publication or the company. If I was going to talk, I really wanted to use that shoot as an example of a wider issue, not an excuse to point the finger at one magazine.

During the interview, I explained that the whole experience had really opened my eyes to just how much our entire world is curated. It wasn't just the billboards and the magazines any more, I'd realised, but the things we see and show of ourselves on the phones we hold in our hands every day. People have the ability, with a click of a button, to alter their own appearance through apps like Facetune or with special preset filters for use on social media. It's no longer just the high-end photo shoots that are fooling us, but the girl we follow on Instagram who posts a photo of herself sitting in a cafe with slightly whitened teeth and a narrowed waist. Retouching is everywhere. It's hidden in plain sight. Right from the minute we wake up to the minute we turn off our phones at night, we are subconsciously being fed the message that we aren't good enough.

How can we expect to look in the mirror and be content with what we see when our phones offer an edited, 'perfected' image of both ourselves and other people? Reality will never compare with that.

'So what's the solution?' the journalist asked me at the end of the interview.

> Retouching is everywhere. It's hidden in plain sight. Right from the minute we wake up to the minute we turn off our phones at night, we are subconsciously being fed the message that we aren't good enough.

I hadn't planned my answers (for most interviews, I don't), so I simply said, 'I just feel like there needs to be some label that tells us whether an image has been photoshopped. A disclosure. Like a warning on a cigarette packet saying, "This may harm your health."'

A MONTH LATER, THE most incredible thing happened. The same company that had photoshopped my images reached out to ask if I'd like to be on the front cover of another one of their magazines. This time, they said, they wanted me to front a campaign that was fully photoshop-free.

Of course I agreed — this is how we create change — and when I got the images back I shared one on Instagram with the following caption:

> Recently I spoke out against images of me being photoshopped and a month later here I am on my first magazine cover 100 per cent as me, and I could not be prouder if I tried.
>
> It just doesn't make sense that we are trying to preach to young girls to be comfortable in their skin yet images of people are still being manipulated in magazines or in the media or on social media to look somewhat 'perfect'. I think it's time we stop and ask ourselves why. Why are we pushing for this unattainable beauty? Why are we trying to fool people into thinking people are something other than what they are?
>
> It would be BONKERS for me to photoshop a real leg onto my fake leg to hide what makes me unique, right? So why are we photoshopping people to remove the things that make them human?!

A FEW WEEKS LATER, I heard from the organisers of TEDxAuckland. Did I want to give a talk? Of course I did, and in the ten days they gave me I came up with a presentation that I titled 'Unreality: Why are we chasing an unachievable idea of perfection?' (And yes, before you ask, 2018 was an incredible but non-stop year — I get exhausted even reflecting on it!) In the space of twelve minutes on the TEDx stage, I told my story and explained why I felt we needed a disclosure on advertising to tell us when something had been retouched. 'Young people don't grow up hating their bodies,' I said. 'It's something we teach them to do.'

TED's slogan is 'ideas worth spreading', and I left the stage that day hoping someone in a position of power would pick up my idea and spread it. In the meantime, I figured that the best I could do was to keep talking about it and encouraging the change that needed to happen.

But I woke up a couple of mornings later and thought, *Why am I waiting for someone else to do this? Why can't I be the person to do it?*

So I sent Brooke a text message: 'Hey, how do I go about talking to someone about getting a law put in place?'

He replied moments later: 'I'll text Jacinda Ardern.'

I a thousand per cent thought he was joking. There was no way he was actually going to text the prime minister.

Next thing I knew, he sent me back a screenshot. It was a

message from Jacinda Ardern herself. Only in New Zealand! In summary, she recommended I start a petition. So I went straight to my desk, sat down and googled 'how to start a petition in NZ'. It didn't take long to work it all out, and I'd soon set up a petition calling for a law to be passed that all commercially used images must have a disclosure if the model has been photoshopped. Then I posted the link to social media, asking people to sign it.

Before long, I got a call from the *New Zealand Herald*. They wanted to do a photo shoot and a write-up on my petition.

'Of course,' I said. 'On one condition: no photoshop.'

The day the paper came out, I spotted it when I went to grab a coffee from my local cafe. It was pretty hard to miss: there was my face on the front page, beneath the headline 'Model vs Photoshop — "There's no need at all".'

And just like that, something that had been little more than a passing idea in response to a journalist's question became something real and massive. Soon, I had appeared on current affairs shows across New Zealand and Australia, and publications worldwide were talking about my petition. I decided I wanted to get to 10,000 signatures, as with that amount it would have to be considered by Parliament. Go big or go home, I figured.

The questions I got from the various shows and publications I spoke to were pretty eye-opening. I was asked more than once, and always by men, how photoshopping an image is any different from wearing make-up. In response, I simply asked them to think specifically about the world they would want their children to grow up in. Sure, the make-up conversation is an interesting one — where *do* we draw the line? But make-up is a tool that people can choose to use, if they want to, to enhance their existing features. Image retouching, on the other hand, is a tool that's used to change someone's appearance completely, and often regardless of whether that person or model wants it or not.

That's also the thing about change, isn't it? In order to get to the place we need to be, we often have to go through a change that feels uncomfortable.

I also had well-known presenters telling me before interviews, 'Ah, you're so brave choosing not to have your images photoshopped. I much prefer when they fix mine up.' I would just smile politely. There wasn't really anything to say to that. Some battles are bigger than small chat. And that's also the thing about change, isn't it? In order to get to the place we need to be, we often have to go through a change that feels uncomfortable.

With every interview, I gained more drive to keep advocating and keep gathering signatures. I found myself repeatedly doing photo shoots with brands that also wanted to take a stand against image retouching, and I had countless conversations with others that wanted to know how they could be a part of the change. That was when I realised that getting these brands on board because they wanted the change was actually going to be more powerful than forcing them to change because of a law.

It had become about so much more than just my petition.

IT WAS DURING THIS time that I made the decision to really throw myself into modelling. It was a massive leap, but one of the best ways for me to get my message out there. Instead of just advocating for more realness in the images we're shown, I knew I also needed to be the change I wanted to see.

In 2019, I was signed to another modelling agency, BELLA in Australia. One of the first things they asked me to do was fly over to walk the runway during Melbourne Fashion Week. I agreed, even though it was so far outside of my comfort zone. The hard part about modelling for me is the way my body functions — or sometimes doesn't. Some pants don't work for me, I struggle with most shoes, and I can move at only one pace. Walking down a runway in unfamiliar shoes and clothes in front of an international audience? Absolutely terrifying. But it was an opportunity to make a stand, literally. I had never walked an international

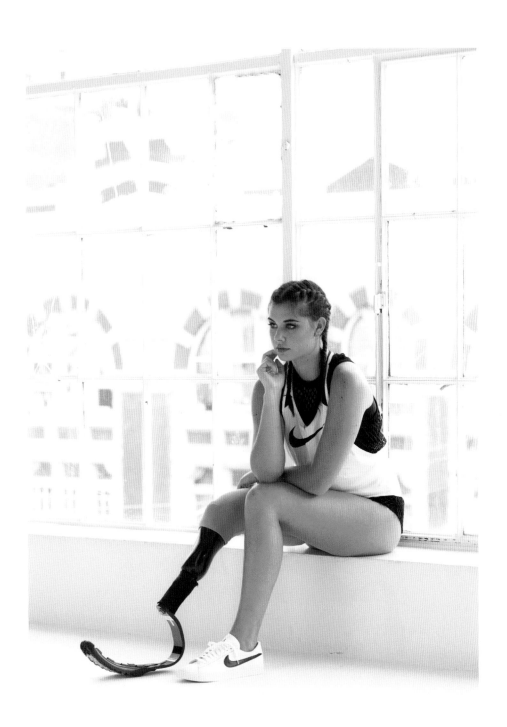

An image from the 2016 photo shoot that went viral. The pics were taken by my photographer friend Jono Parker and it was my first try at modelling.

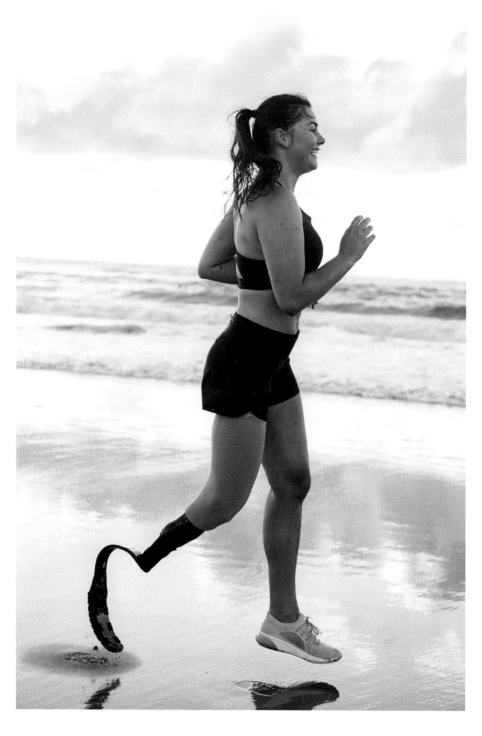

Striding down the beach on a modelling assignment for activewear company Athleta in Sydney, 2018. I love this photo because it captures how happy I was in that moment, just enjoying moving my body. PHOTO BY BEAU GREALY

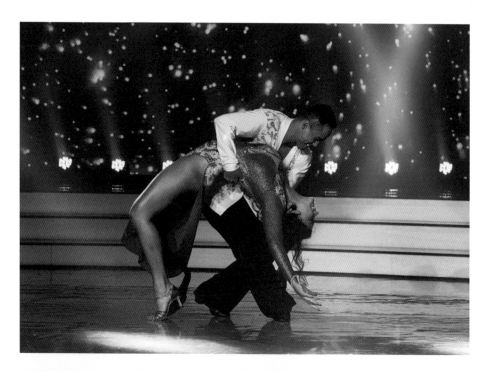

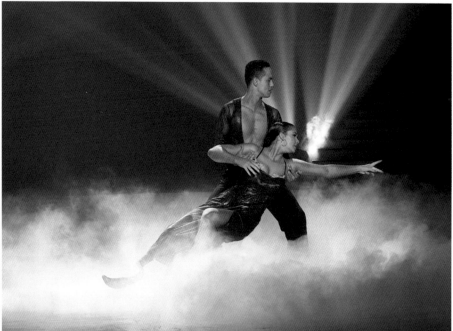

Top
Performing my first dance with partner Jonny Williams on *Dancing with the Stars*, May 2018.

Bottom
Dancing with Jonny in the grand final, July 2018. We placed third overall.

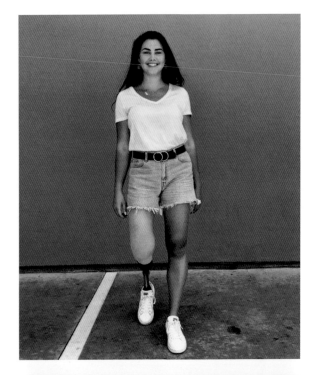

Right
One of my first shoots
with Natural Models LA
in August 2018.

Below
Modelling in the Jockey show
at New Zealand Fashion
Week, 30 August 2018.
PHOTO BY STEFAN GOSATTI/
GETTY IMAGES

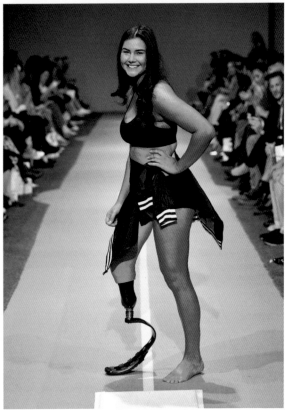

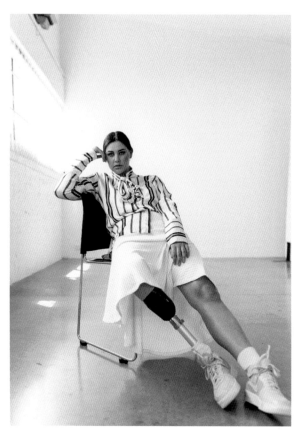

Two favourite images from a studio shoot with talented New Zealand photographer Brijana Cato, December 2018.

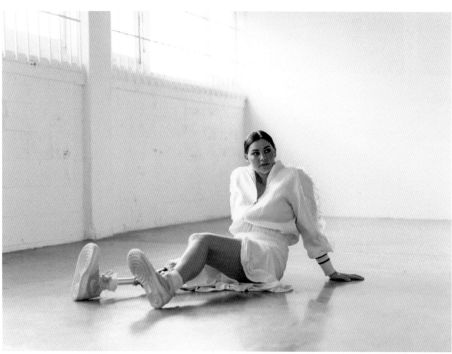

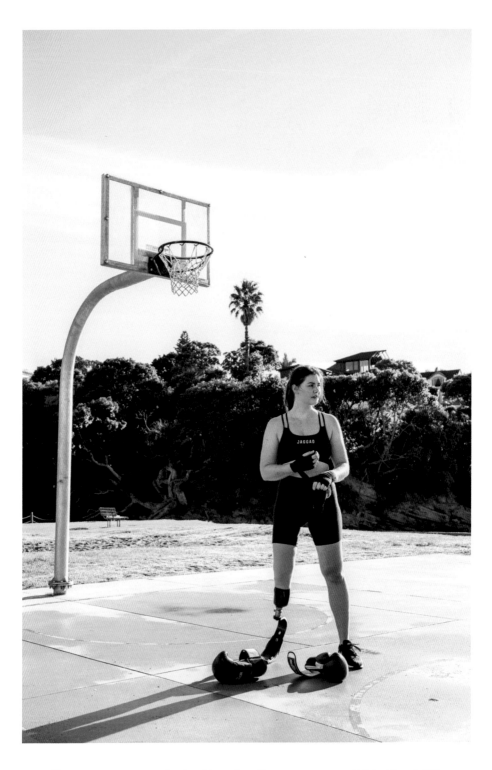

Shooting a campaign for health and wellbeing company AIA in May 2019,
after I became one of their AIA Vitality ambassadors.

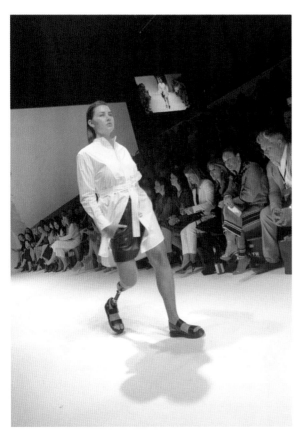

Left
Stepping outside my comfort zone to walk the runway at Melbourne Fashion Week, July 2019.

Below
Quad biking at Joshua Tree National Park in California in December 2019: a great way to cap off a full-on year.

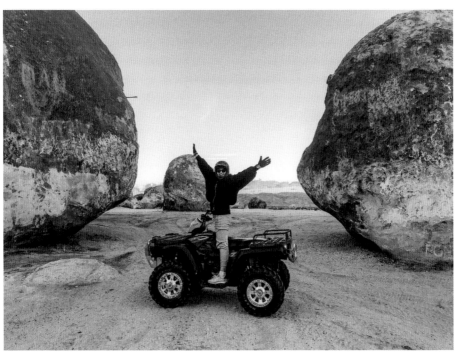

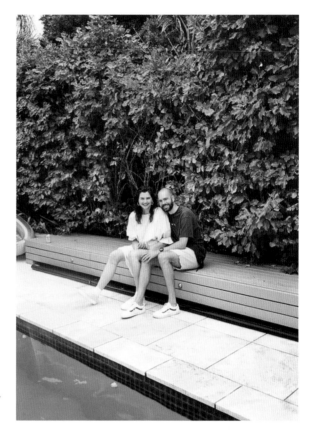

Right
Hanging by the pool with
my partner, Todd, during
Christmas 2020 celebrations.

Below
Having a cuddle with
my dog Scout, 2021.

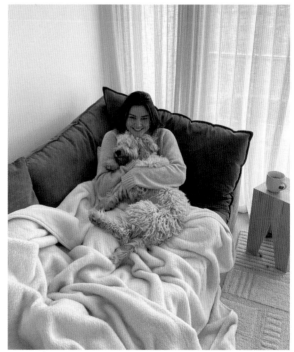

runway before, but I kept telling myself that if I could dance live on TV then I could definitely do this.

I was also asked to be an ambassador for Melbourne Fashion Week, and invited to speak on a panel about diversity and inclusion alongside Chelsea Bonner, the founder of BELLA, and Robyn Lawley, an incredible curve model. The three of us talked about how the world has made some good steps towards more diversity and inclusion, but pointed out that we still have so far to go. You can see that in the fact that we live in a world where people are afraid to leave the house without make-up on or won't post to social media without hiding their real face beneath a filter. The idea of tokenism came up more than once, especially how you will often arrive at a shoot and discover you're the only 'plus-size' or 'diverse' model there. On the one hand it's disheartening because it feels like you're just there to help the brand tick a box, but on the flip side you also hope that your presence will bring at least some change regardless of the brand's intent. Interestingly, that was exactly the case with the runway show I walked in — it was incredible, but I definitely stood out as the token diversity model. Despite that, I do believe change has to start somewhere, and if it was going to happen anywhere then this was it.

After every photo shoot I do or runway I walk, I get a flood of messages thanking me for showing different bodies in our world. That in itself is enough to keep me going. I also think I might have been told I'm an inspiration more times in my life than I've been called my own name. Honestly, that always makes me a bit uncomfortable, because I'm actually not a huge fan of attention (despite my job). At the same time, though, it does make me feel warm inside — I mean, what an honour it is to be a small shaft of light in someone else's life.

Why is it exactly that when I step out in the body I call home I'm inspirational, but when my sisters do the same thing it's barely noteworthy?

Inspiration is an interesting one. There's a whole conversation to be had there. I'm often asked for my thoughts on what's dubbed 'inspiration porn' — the concept that we put people who are 'different' or speaking their truth on pedestals because we think they're brave for showing their true self — and it's something I've avoided talking about until now. It has always felt a little weird to me that I can post a photo of myself walking down the beach in a bikini and instantly be flooded with 'you're so inspiring' comments. Meanwhile, my sisters, both small able-bodied fair-skinned women, could post the exact same style of photo and get zero comments that mention inspiration. Why is it exactly that when I step out in the body I call home I'm inspirational, but when my sisters do the same thing it's barely noteworthy? I am just doing what they're doing. I'm just out here living my life with what I have.

Sometimes I wonder what people expect me to do. Sure, I've been given a rough hand. Most days it crosses my mind that I wish certain things were easier, that I didn't have to think about all of the things I do have to think about. But this is the hand I was dealt. Yeah, it's hard, but at the end of the day it's the life I have and I get only one chance at it. So I'm going to push through the hard days to make the most of what I'm given. I want to be here, I want to experience everything this world has to offer, and I want to do it while I can — because who knows what's next? No matter how hard things get, there is still so much good to be found. You just have to choose to see it.

This plays into the bigger need to keep normalising our different bodies and different experiences. Being able to find inspiration in something or someone is hugely important. It's one of the ways we motivate each other to be better and do better, but the thing I've always wondered is this: why is someone standing confidently in their skin an inspiration? Maybe it's simply because, for too long, we've been given only the narrowest view of what a 'normal' human looks like, so anything that sits outside of that is 'different'. We then find solace in an image of someone who is 'different', but the fact is that anyone who's raw and vulnerable and honest is actually more closely linked to us than we might realise. Sure, they're 'different' from what we've been led to believe is the norm — but they are actually far closer to who we are. Our differences are the things that unite us. The more we can each be vulnerable and show up in our unique bodies with our unique life experiences, the more we will start to see inspiration as 'normal'. And maybe, just maybe, we will start to see inspiration within ourselves.

The only real difference between you and me isn't that I'm inspiring. It's simply that I found out really young exactly how brave and strong I am because life put me to the test.

You are strong too — so much stronger than you even know. If you haven't faced that test yet, don't wait for it.

Be your own inspiration.

Get out there and live your best damn life.

A MONTH AFTER MELBOURNE Fashion Week, I got a huge job for a well-known lingerie brand in Sydney. It was a two-day shoot alongside two other models, none of the images would be photoshopped, and the campaign would be shown in store windows across Australia and New Zealand.

It was another one of those pinch-me experiences. Here I was, the same person who as a young girl had spent years trying to cover up her body, about to be shown in her underwear on store billboards across two countries.

I instantly thought of that young girl walking to school. *This is the moment*, I thought.

The images went live in stores at the end of the year, and a few weeks later I got the following direct message on Instagram.

> Hey, Jess,
>
> Just wanted to say I was in the mall the other day with Miss Nine. She looked up at the poster and said, 'Mum, look it's Jess.'
>
> I said, 'Yeah, hunny, it is. Doesn't she look amazing?'
>
> She looked at me and said, 'Mum, we all look amazing and Jess is just being herself.'
>
> I looked and said, 'And what is that?'
>
> She said, 'Natural and beautiful all wrapped up together.'
>
> So thank you for being you and allowing a nine-year-old to comment on us being amazing.

That young girl I'd imagined for so many years walking home from school? She was real. Miss Nine. And she had seen me on a billboard, and she had understood that different is normal.

If that's not a dream come true, I don't know what is.

9

Facing the storm

There's just one problem with writing the story of your life. While you're writing, life keeps happening. And if I've learnt anything from my life up until this point, it's that you can never be sure what's waiting around the next corner. Life is always a work in progress.

To be honest, I don't even want to write the chapter you're about to read. I don't know where to start, and I definitely don't have an ending. It could be summed up in one sentence: I didn't climb a mountain to be defeated by this hill. But shit, has it tested my patience.

Shall we leave it at that?

OF COURSE, I'M NOT going to leave it at that. It wouldn't be true Jess Quinn style not to ramble the full story, piece by piece, until you and I both have the full picture. But here's the basic version: the past few years have tested me more than anything else in my life. As what had been my most incredible year ever drew to a close, everything started to fall apart.

When I came off *Dancing with the Stars* in August 2018, I was blown away by how well my body had adapted to and endured the physical strain it had faced. I'd done the same amount of training in three months that I would normally have done over two years, and I'd done almost all of it on one leg. My prosthetic side had handled it amazingly well, while my good leg hadn't flared up at all. The only thing that had really gone wrong was my broken rib, but in all honesty it was nice to have an injury that didn't involve unanswered questions or a backwards foot.

Then, one night in November, I was sitting at home on the couch when, out of the blue, I noticed that the inner thigh of my good leg was incredibly swollen. When I touched it, it was sore, and I could feel some sort of lump. As anyone who has had cancer will know, the sudden discovery of an unexplained lump can cause an overwhelming amount of anxiety. I tried not to worry about it too much, and pushed it to the back of my mind, hoping it would just go away on its own.

As anyone who has had cancer will know, the sudden discovery of an unexplained lump can cause an overwhelming amount of anxiety.

Then, a few days later, my left foot started to feel really unusual — numb, tingly and incredibly heavy. I wasn't really sure whether it was an actual physical symptom or something I was imagining out of fear, but I decided I'd better take myself to the doctor for peace of mind. Before I knew it, I found myself at the hospital, hooked up to IV lines and being put through a series of tests. The doctors initially suspected I might have a blood clot in my leg. They also checked for tumours and documented all my symptoms. Then they sent my tests off and we waited for the results.

My mum's face the next day when the doctor came in and ruled out any form of cancer was enough to make me never want to tell her I'd been admitted to hospital ever again. I can't imagine the fear my parents must hold around me getting sick again. Sure, it scares me, but not as much as it must scare them. They saw and understood so much more than I did back when I was a child.

I felt a sense of relief knowing nothing sinister was lurking beneath my skin, but there was also the familiar frustration of having to walk away with no answers.

I spent five days in the hospital, long enough for pretty much everything to be ruled out and nothing to be found except a very minor crossover of my veins. The doctors thought this might potentially be causing a blood-flow issue, but said that was very unlikely.

They told me to keep an eye out for certain symptoms, then sent me on my way.

I felt a sense of relief knowing nothing sinister was lurking beneath my skin, but there was also the familiar frustration of having to walk away with no answers. That's always been much worse for me, and it's something I've learnt is part and parcel of living in a body that's so vastly different from most. As I've said, I've never had a how-to guide or a big group of people to compare notes with. I'm basically trying to navigate the world solo.

Once I got home from the hospital, I made the decision to stop training for a while. After years of intense exercise and months of dancing, my body was clearly screaming out for a break. I had no desire to push it and risk harming the only good leg I have left. So I stopped going to the gym, stopped walking, stopped doing workouts at home. I went from being incredibly active to doing almost nothing.

A FEW MONTHS LATER, in early 2019, I headed over to Italy for a work trip. It wasn't my first time in Europe. Four years earlier, I'd gone on a three-month OE, starting with a five-week tour with a bunch of other travellers I'd never met before through something like sixteen different countries, and ending with some time in London and Greece with some friends from home.

Honestly, thinking about that trip and how carefree I was still blows my mind. The tour was an incredible experience, but it wasn't without its challenges. One day while in Croatia, I was rushing to get ready for dinner (everything on that tour was fast-paced) and went to take a shower in the poky hostel bathroom. When I got out and went to put my leg on, I noticed that one of the straps had fallen off — at the time, my prosthetic was done up with two

Velcro straps instead of a corset, and I needed both straps to make it fit properly. I went and told the tour manager, and he came with me — while everyone else went off and had dinner — to wander around the small town we were in, trying to find a prosthetic shop that could fix my leg. No one could understand what we were trying to say, even when we spoke in the simplest terms, and we didn't know a word of Croatian. In the end, I had to rely on Kiwi ingenuity: when we found a hardware store, I bought some cable ties and used those to tie my leg on.

On that trip, I walked all day, every day, and I never remember my leg getting sore once, but when I returned to Italy in 2019 I felt a bit nervous. I knew there would be lots of walking involved, but while resting and recovering with my injured leg I'd gone from my usual 10,000-plus steps a day to somewhere closer to 4000.

In the end, I had to rely on Kiwi ingenuity: when we found a hardware store, I bought some cable ties and used those to tie my leg on.

Well, on my first day in Italy I managed to walk 11,000 steps while exploring the city. Since I'd first discovered the swelling in my groin back in November, I'd been tracking what I called #healtheleg on Instagram, so people could follow along with my rehab journey. Just before I'd left New Zealand, I'd discovered I actually had a torn adductor — the muscles that sit around your hips — on that side, and things had finally begun to settle after some rehab. At the end of that first day in Italy, I posted a photo with the caption: 'This is the face of a human that walked 11,000 steps today. Is #healtheleg heading towards #healedtheleg? I think YES.'

But the very next morning, I woke up and found that my other foot — as in, the backwards one — had swollen up so badly I couldn't get my prosthetic on. Any change in the shape or form of my foot means the prosthetic won't fit, so I had some ice delivered to my room, then sat out on the balcony in the cold, hoping the ice and the freezing air would bring my foot back down to a more normal size. This new swelling looked like I had a tight rubber band across the arch of my foot and everything below it had blown up.

To be honest, I was less stressed about my swollen foot than I was about making sure I could attend my four jam-packed days of work. I simply figured that the swelling would, like most obstacles, sort itself out. And after two long-haul flights and another shorter one, a bit of swelling wasn't overly surprising. I eventually managed to get my prosthetic on, but I had to go through the same ice-and-balcony routine every morning I was in Italy before I could head out to work.

Afterwards, I flew on to Los Angeles for another month of work there. I was still waiting on my visa, but making regular trips to the States in the meantime to try to get the ball rolling. While I was there, the swelling in my right foot kept coming and going, but I figured it was just another bump in the road. I stuck with ice, lying on the floor with my legs up the wall and rest, and somehow made it to all of my work commitments.

Once I was back home, though, the swelling on my right side was still causing me trouble. It was almost as if #healtheleg had decided to swap from one leg to another. After one especially difficult weekend, I posted a photo to Instagram of myself sitting in bed with my prosthetic off, and the following caption beneath:

Saturday was not a good day.

If you've been following me for a while, you'll probably know that, as well as the injury in my 'good leg', I've been struggling with swelling in what I have left of my other leg. I've been fighting through it for a few months. Most mornings I have to jam my prosthetic on and deal with an hour of not being able to walk well before the swelling goes down (or maybe it becomes numb enough for me to walk on it).

Saturday I woke up and literally could not put

my leg on. I iced, did legs up the wall, then tried again. Still I couldn't put my leg on. So I spent the day in bed feeling very frustrated with life.

Honestly, I'm very over these constant injuries, and not being able to put on my leg was an all-new low. I've always trained and made it my mission to feel strong and able, but lately I've been chasing my tail with setback after setback. But I'm starting to think maybe this is the season for another kind of strength. Maybe life is testing my mental strength and, I can tell ya, it's testing!

But they say nothing goes away until it has taught us what we need to know. So, I'm trying to be patient, trying to stay positive, trying to not let it consume me, reminding myself I will get back to where I was, but it's frustrating, it's hard and THAT'S OKAY. Not every part of life is rainbows and flowers. We need the bad to see the good. Know that it's okay to be angry, it's okay to get mad, to kick and scream. Just try to not unpack and live there.

OF COURSE, THIS WAS all happening just as my career was skyrocketing. As 2018 moved into 2019, I found myself getting all sorts of incredible opportunities, all over the world. I'd also got a book contract, and as I flew from one place to another I started writing down my story. These were the sorts of opportunities I'd once only dreamt of.

Everything I had worked so hard for was finally taking flight, and from the outside my life was incredible — but I was living in a body that seemed to have other ideas. It just didn't want to play ball.

As I've mentioned, I flew to Australia for Melbourne Fashion Week — leaving a day early, in fact, so that I'd have time to ice my leg before I had to walk down the runway — then jetted to Sydney for lingerie shoots, and all the while I was pushing my petition and advocating for realness and diversity in what we're shown. At the same time, I'd almost got my visa for the States, so I'd decided to officially make the move to LA at the end of the year. Everything I had worked so hard for was finally taking flight, and from the outside my life was incredible — but I was living in a body that seemed to have other ideas. It just didn't want to play ball. I have never been one to put my life on hold, though, so I did my best to keep going. I wasn't going to let this bump in the road stop me from achieving the things I had been working towards. I felt I had come too far for that.

I tried to remind myself that this challenge was just

another bout of turbulence. It was making me stronger, bit by bit, even if sometimes I felt like it was doing the opposite. Sometimes the turbulence would be more than I could bear, but I'd remind myself that was okay too. I knew I had everything within me I needed in order to survive. One thing I have learnt by now is that setbacks don't have to be overcome. Adversity happens. There's nothing you can do about that. What you can do is find a way to live through it and live with it. You can be struggling and still live your life. Things can be really hard at the same time as they're really good. The key is finding a way to adapt, to let both the adversity and life's gifts in at the same time. Because in between all the hard moments, especially the ones that go on longer than you expect, are the incredible things that happen — the new relationships and friends and family members, the exciting opportunities, the sunrises, the sunsets, the belly laughs. Whenever I look back on a storm I've already survived, I question whether it was actually as big or intense as it seemed at the time. With hindsight, I can see it was just a moment of bad weather that was inevitably broken by more sunshine. So I always try to remember that, even if I don't know when or how, this storm too will pass.

I guess what I am trying to say is that this life isn't easy — not at all — but that's okay. It's not about living a life without knocks and scars.

It's about living a life full stop.

IN A MATTER OF months, #healtheleg somehow became a story of healing two legs. The ongoing swelling in my right foot caused me to lean even more heavily than usual on my left leg, and that just caused my groin injury to flare up again. After I'd discovered the tear in my left adductor, my physio worked out that a bunch of other stuff was going and making things worse too. As per usual with me, it was the opposite of simple. Before the swelling in my right leg began in Italy, my groin had felt like it was settling — but I soon realised that the injury on that side had just been lying dormant before it began getting worse again.

It was the swelling on the right side, though, that was the biggest concern for me. That was the main thing holding me back, the thing that I just couldn't find any answers for. Google wasn't much help — you try searching for 'swelling in backwards foot' and see what you get. Even a search for 'rotationplasty swelling' doesn't go so well — it comes up with explanations of what rotationplasty is. I had spent years coming to terms with just how unique my body is in a visual sense, but now I had to navigate that uniqueness from an entirely functional perspective.

The first person I went to see was Mike, my surgeon. He's still my first port of call whenever something goes wrong with my leg. He ordered X-rays and scans, and confirmed that everything was looking okay mechanically.

I then explored every other area possible. I went to see

countless specialists. Every appointment took twice as long as it might have, because the specialist would have never seen anyone like me. Before they could even begin to try to work out whether they could do anything to help, they would first have to get over their obvious excitement at seeing such a medical rarity. Some specialists or practitioners were so totally unequipped to deal with such a unique body that they would just stare blankly. Sometimes, I've found it quite cool to be such a rarity — as much as it's hard, it's also awesome to be in a body so miraculous.

Every appointment took twice as long as it might have, because the specialist would have never seen anyone like me.

This was not one of those times. Now, I wanted nothing more than to be following in the footsteps of thousands of others with similar experiences. I wanted there to be a straightforward answer.

But every specialist would bump me along to another. I went to lymphatic specialists and vascular specialists, I got all sorts of tests done, I tried all sorts of devices and creams and treatments. Every time I walked into a new clinic, I would be filled with hope.

This is it, I would think. *This is the place where I'll find the answer I need.*

It never was. I would just leave with more frustration and less money in the bank.

I even contacted the few people I could find online from around the world who'd had a rotationplasty. Had they experienced anything similar? None of them had. And even if they did mention that they'd had swelling too, I'd discover that their experiences and lives were so vastly different from mine that it was pretty much impossible to gain any guidance there. It was one big guessing game.

Every test came back clear and without answers, and every day I woke up with a swollen red foot that wouldn't go into my prosthetic. I would ice it, put my legs up the wall, take a cold shower, jam it into my prosthetic and limp around home for an hour until I could do a movement that somewhat replicated walking. Then I would leave the house to attend physio, acupuncture, the chiropractor and whatever other appointments I had. At the end of the day, I would get home and struggle to pull my prosthetic off because my foot had swollen to the point where it was almost stuck. When I removed my foot, it was only to find that it looked as if it had been stung by a bee. Then the next day I would get up and do it all over again. It was relentless.

I got so frustrated I remember thinking, *If someone told me there was a secondary cancer in there, I would be relieved*, then instantly felt guilty for even having the thought. I would never wish to go through that again, but I just really wanted an answer as to why I was in so much pain and discomfort.

I wanted to know why, all of a sudden, my life had changed pace.

AS THE MONTHS WORE on and the #healtheleg saga continued, it got harder and harder to keep going. There were times when I would spend days prepping for a speaking engagement, only to wake up on the morning of the event and find I was unable to put my leg on. I'd have to call Brooke, then head back to bed while he tried to find someone to replace me at short notice. I hate letting people down more than anything. Not only had I been forced to give up the training I loved so much, but now I was having to cancel on the work I'd spent so long chasing.

But, after years of having people constantly worrying about me, I have developed an incredible talent for throwing on a smile and pretending everything is okay. I'm so good at it, I often fool myself. So, for the most part, that's what I did — I didn't let people in on exactly how bad things were. I shared some of what I was going through with #healtheleg, but I kept the worst of it behind closed doors. I preferred to step out of the house (when it was physically possible) with a smile on my face. Call it a coping mechanism. It's my way of ensuring I don't get stuck in a place I can't get out of. It's my way of surviving everything I've been through without allowing it to take a greater toll on me than it must. I don't like making a fuss, I don't like putting people out and I detest sympathy, so I would go along to my work commitments with a leg that felt like it was about to explode out of my prosthetic, and no one would know. I've never found any comfort in the sympathy I get handed when I ask for help — it's like nails down a chalkboard to me, and just makes me feel uncomfortable and inadequate. Is this something I should unpack? Probably. But it's just how I am.

So I persevered, smiling outwardly, while still searching high and low for answers. Once I'd covered off and cleared any potential medical conditions, I started to explore whether it might be something my prosthetic itself was triggering. I went to the Limb Centre and showed them my swollen red foot, but again they'd never seen anything like it. I was the first person like me they'd ever built a prosthetic for, so it was all new territory. The usual story. They shaved some of the inside of my prosthetic leg socket to make a bit more space for my foot, and while that helped a bit at first, ultimately it just gave my leg more space to swell. So I took my search overseas and spent the best bit of half a year reaching out and talking to people from around the world about whether they could help. Every lead ran dry. No one seemed to have any advice. No one had any ideas about what I could do.

With every dead end and every morning that I woke up to a foot that wouldn't go into my prosthetic, I sank deeper into a hole. My issues with my legs were affecting everything in my life, but sometimes you don't realise you're falling until you hit the ground. I began to notice I lacked my usual motivation. I wasn't my usual upbeat self. I started making excuses for not doing the things I love — things like my work or spending time with friends. Although I knew these things would probably give me the distraction I needed, I just felt like I didn't have the mental capacity for anything more than dealing with my legs.

Sometimes you don't realise you're falling until you hit the ground. I began to notice I lacked my usual motivation. I wasn't my usual upbeat self. I started making excuses for not doing the things I love.

I began asking myself questions I have never wanted to ask. Questions like, *What happens if my legs don't get better? Will I be able to live the life I've imagined?*

I had thoughts I've never wanted to think, like wishing so badly I was living in a different body.

I felt emotions I've never wanted to feel, including the sort of total exhaustion that comes not from needing to sleep but from having no idea how much longer you can keep getting out of bed with a smile on your face.

I relived moments I never wanted to experience again.

I felt as though I had completely lost myself and everything I had worked for years to gain.

I lost myself while trying to find answers.

I lost hope.

While I was going through all of this, I was also busy trying to write this book, and I started questioning why I was even bothering. In fact, this book took much longer to arrive in your hands than I'd originally hoped because of all of this. Sitting and trying to write about all the times that were so positive and great while I was struggling to even look at the leg I have left was one of the most challenging things I've ever had to do. At times, I considered just taking a match to these pages and setting them all alight. As I wrote about all the things I've worked so hard for, all the things I've said and done, I found myself questioning whether the life I've lived was ever a reality, whether anything I've felt for the majority of my life is even true. It began to feel fraudulent to claim it was, given the reality I was living felt so vastly different. I've always said that, given the opportunity, I wouldn't change what I went through — but how could I write those words when what I found myself feeling was the exact opposite?

And here is the whole truth of it: while you'll finish this chapter in a few pages, it's not actually over yet for me. I'm still in it. This is still my life. I don't know when this chapter is going to end for me. Over the past few years, each mountain has led directly to another mountain with tougher terrain. It feels like I'm constantly fighting an uphill battle.

This is the darkness I've been living in for the past few years. It might be only a fraction of time compared with the rest of my life, but more than once it has been completely overwhelming. It has overshadowed all of the good stuff. And when I realised that, I knew I needed to write about this more than ever.

This is still my life. I don't know when this chapter is going to end for me. Over the past few years, each mountain has led directly to another mountain with tougher terrain. It feels like I'm constantly fighting an uphill battle.

Because isn't this true for all of us?

You can have an absolutely amazing day, then one bad thing happens and all of a sudden you've forgotten every good thing that came before it and will come after. You start to believe that the one bad moment was actually a whole bad day — and if you don't manage to get out of that space, then all of a sudden you're thinking you've had a bad week, a bad month, a bad year.

I've always felt called to speak honestly about just how

hard things get, because that's always been my reality. That means speaking up when things truly are at their hardest. I have always known that mine isn't the easy path, but for most of my life post-cancer the hurdles I've faced have been manageable, especially when compared with everything I've already been through. But they aren't manageable any more. They're totally out of my control. They feel, at times, entirely insurmountable.

While I hope that this chapter of my life will one day be merely that — a moment in time when things weren't great — I can't tell you that yet. I simply have no idea when this particular storm will end, or how. This might just be my life now. This might be how my body works. Maybe the window of my life where I lived actively and carefree with my prosthetic has closed.

I just don't know.

That's the challenge of living in this body.

This is the mountain I'm climbing now.

It's one of the first times in my life when I've had to stop many times along the way, when I've contemplated going back down to the bottom, when I've been forced to retreat a bit so that I can have another go.

But one thing I do know: I am yet to meet a mountain I can't climb.

I know I'm a match for my mountains.

I've got this — even when I feel like I don't.

COME NOVEMBER 2019, I was living between LA and Auckland. I should have been living the dream, but I wasn't. I was living in a body I didn't want to be in.

The cruel irony, of course, is that this body of mine, the thing that was keeping me from my dreams, was also the thing that had got me to this place in my career. I'd spent years sharing my story, showcasing my difference to the world, achieving things I'd never thought possible, all in an attempt to get exactly where I was, and it was this body that carried me through all of that. It's what helped me grow into the person I am. It's what enabled me to do all of those things. But then it suddenly flipped and became the thing that was inhibiting me from enjoying the same opportunities it had offered me not long before. On the one hand, this unique body of mine had created all of these opportunities, then on the other it became the barrier to me taking any of them.

With my move to LA, my original dream — the one of being on a billboard so I could normalise different — was materialising right before my eyes. I was getting opportunity after opportunity — not only to be on billboards, but also in storefronts and magazines and advertising campaigns. But I often had to turn down these opportunities because I knew my body simply wasn't up to the task. I had to balance any shoots I did attend with days afterwards in bed nursing a swollen leg. For the most part, I pushed through physically, but mentally it started to feel impossible. I no longer enjoyed doing any of these things because of the price I'd have to pay in the hours and days afterwards. Don't get me wrong, it was still always worth it when I saw the impact of the end result. But when I read all the messages of love I received from people all over the world, I'd inevitably be doing it in bed, covered with ice packs.

It just seemed so unfair.

I've always been an incredibly positive person, and on the outside I still was — but, on the inside, I realised I was speaking to myself in a way I would never speak to anyone else.

One thing I've rarely struggled with in life is my mental health, but living with this pain and uncertainty for so long weighed on me, to the point that it ended up affecting my state of mind. I became unhappy, and I began to lose myself. I was taken right back to when I was younger and lay in bed crying every night, asking, 'Why me?' My internal dialogue became something I didn't like. I've always been an incredibly positive person, and on the outside I still was — but, on the inside, I realised I was speaking to myself in a way I would never speak to anyone else. I knew what was happening in my mind was situational, a product of what

I was going through, but since I had no control over the situation that knowledge didn't really help. To add to it all, I couldn't even go and get the endorphin kick I usually would from moving my body and working out. At first it was okay, because I kept telling myself this would all end, just like every other hiccup in my life. But the longer it went on, the more I questioned whether it actually would.

The toll that living in pain takes on your mental health is huge.

The toll of constantly trying to find answers for something, only to be constantly left wondering, is huge.

The toll of waking up and not knowing whether or not you can live the day you had planned because it all depends on whether or not you can don a body part is huge.

I was living with all of that.

The stress of it all was exhausting. Living in a body that doesn't do the things your mind wants to do. The constant mental battle over whether to keep trying or to give up and accept that this was my lot. The questions that rolled around and around in my mind: *Maybe I just need to let it all go? Maybe if I push through, the pain and discomfort will disappear? Maybe it's all in my head?*

For the first time in my life post-cancer, I felt truly disabled by my body. I found myself struggling to do so many things that I was forced to confront my feelings about the word 'disability' all over again. This time, though, I had to do it after some of the most super-abled years I'd ever lived. Part of me felt an immense sense of guilt. Maybe I'd just been hiding from my disability? Maybe this was my body telling me that, no matter how hard I tried, I wasn't as able as I wished I was? Another part of me, realising that I simply couldn't keep going at the same pace as I had been for the past decade, was overcome with an immense sense of defeat.

Being as able as I possibly can be has always been my main goal. I've never wanted what I went through and the body I now live in to dictate who I am or what I can try to do. I've never wanted to live by the dictionary definition of disabled, even if that was how some people might have described my body.

> **Being as able as I possibly can be
> has always been my main goal. I've
> never wanted what I went through
> and the body I now live in to dictate
> who I am or what I can try to do.**

I've always told myself I'm not wounded, lame, hurt, wrecked, sidelined, helpless, incapable or powerless. So what, I lost a leg? I've spent years refusing to let that get in my way. Year by year, challenge by challenge, I've found a way to write my own definition for the body I live in.

But then life handed me this particular challenge and, for the first time since I was a young kid lying in hospital with a cancer that was trying to take over my body, I had to admit that I felt hurt.

I felt wounded.

I felt sidelined.

I felt incapable.

The biggest achievement of my day used to be the 10,000 steps I'd done, or the talk I'd just given to hundreds of people, or the abilities I'd gained while training. Now? My biggest achievement was a day where my leg would actually go on.

I felt helpless.

I felt incredibly powerless.

I grew up in a world that can be really unkind to — or outright disadvantage — people like me. It's a world that isn't made for people like me, a world that doesn't make life easy for people like me, a world that doesn't show people like me as successful and happy. But I wasn't born like this. I lived eight years before I became a person who has different needs from the majority. And, when my body did change, I was never made to feel different. I never felt like I missed out on opportunities. I never felt like I couldn't or shouldn't try to do something, or that I wasn't welcome to try anything or to go anywhere. I never felt marginalised. But a large portion of people like me — people who the world calls 'disabled' — do feel like that. They're not accepted in the way I have been, and for the longest time I had no idea why I was accepted when others weren't. It's only recently that I've learnt that it's because of privilege.

Sure, I'm technically part of a minority group, but every other privilege I have has outweighed the one privilege I don't have: an 'abled' body. Sure, I don't have two legs like most other people, but there's so much else I *do* have. I'm white, so I have all the privileges that come with that — I've never had to deal with discrimination on the grounds of my race. I grew up with, and still have, financial stability. Whether by nature or nurture, I also grew up having the confidence to tell people how I wanted to be treated. I never stood for second best with my prosthetics or my treatments. I never stood for being told I was 'disabled'. I know now that having that confidence is in itself a privilege.

Thanks to the many conversations I've been lucky to have with people whose lived experiences have been so different from my own, I've learnt that the way I've experienced life with a differently abled body is very different from how many others experience it. So many privileges have made my experience, although incredibly difficult, a lot easier than it might have been. Had I not been diagnosed with cancer at eight and had I not lost my leg at nine, I would never have known the hardships of this life I have. I never would have had this first-hand perspective of how having an 'abled' body is a privilege.

Too often, this category of society that I fall into doesn't get a voice. We are an afterthought — an *Oh and we should probably provide ramp access*, a *We are going to have to find a way to include a disabled toilet*. It's like people forget that this could be them. That they, too, are just one unfortunate accident or wrong turn away from joining this group. We're not so far apart from one another's experiences as some might want to think.

There's another thing I have been given: a voice, and a platform where I can make myself heard. And going through all of this, learning all of this, has just made me even more determined than ever to use the platform I have to be a voice for people whose ride has been different from mine, for people who aren't listened to like I am. In saying that, it's not good enough to just hear the voice of one person from a minority and assume that ticks the box. One lone voice does not make a conversation. It doesn't constitute representation.

My difficulties forced me to rethink my relationship with the word 'disability', but this is something we should all be doing. We should all be getting uncomfortable. We should all be learning. And we should see this as a forever project, something we need to keep teaching ourselves and others again and again and again.

THE DIFFERENCE BETWEEN THE time when I first lost my abilities and everything I've gone through with #healtheleg is perspective. The first time round, I was so young, and I spent years regaining my abilities, learning to walk and to move in this new body. These past few years, it's felt like the same thing all over again, but this time I've felt it so much more. This time, I've already spent almost two decades living a life I learnt to love before my abilities were taken away from me. This time, I'm an adult, and fully aware of exactly what I'm missing out on.

The simplest tasks began to feel impossible. Even walking around the supermarket without my leg swelling up so much I couldn't put any weight on it seemed out of reach. Some days I'd wake up, attempt to put my leg on, realise I couldn't and then just get back into bed. And the worst thing about those days? The only thing I *could* do was sit in bed. When you can't put your leg on, basic things like going to the toilet or making lunch are near impossible.

There were moments when, just as I had when I was nine, I would pick up my prosthetic and throw it across my room because I felt so frustrated by everything.

Sometimes, I would actually just allow myself to sit there in bed and be angry. While it was good to let it out, I tried not to do that too often because, inevitably, I would just end up feeling worse. The frustration I felt at my immediate situation would spread to me feeling frustrated about all the things I struggled to do because I couldn't get my leg on.

A lot of people asked me why I didn't just use assistive devices like crutches or a wheelchair on the bad days. I get how that might seem like the easy fix from the outside, but when you've got used to not relying on things like that, suddenly incorporating them can be really challenging. I am also, as you now know, naturally someone who will just persevere. I admit that this might sometimes make things worse. Maybe not putting my leg on for a year could have helped physically. Who knows? Anyway, for a long time after I lost my leg, every goal I set was based on doing things by myself and getting rid of my assistive devices. I still remember the first time I was able to get in and out of the bath without Mum or Dad lifting me. Or the first time I put my shoe on my prosthetic foot without a shoe horn and without my parents helping. Or when, after a decade, I finally threw away the chair I had in the shower because my left leg had become strong enough to stand on without assistance. From that point on, I showered standing on one leg (quite the skill). I saw every one of these things as an achievement — and, in a way, they were.

But the truth is I got to a point where I just didn't even consider assistive devices to be an option. I pushed them away, because I've always wanted to be able to do everything myself. I wanted to do everything like 'everybody else'.

I didn't want to go back to having to rely on any sort of assistive device. It's almost like I thought needing one again would make me weak. But recently, after one too many showers where my good leg felt like it was going to snap because of my groin injury, I ordered myself a new shower chair. For more than a year, I had been thinking about how much it would help me, but I just couldn't bring myself to actually buy it. Eventually, I accepted that spending ten minutes every day standing on a leg that was already injured probably wasn't benefiting my healing. So I got online and ordered the chair, and I couldn't believe the difference it made. I realised that maybe I just need help sometimes, and that's okay.

I posted a picture of my shower chair to Instagram with the following caption.

> I think a lot of us go through life pushing help away. Us humans all live in uniquely different bodies that need help in different ways. There are so many things out there that can make our lives better, or easier, yet we choose not to use them because we're stubborn, or proud, or don't want to seem 'weak'.
>
> Whether it be your mental health or physical health, it's okay to need help. It's okay to ask for assistance. Do the things that will make your life

a little easier, and don't think about what others think or how your life differs from theirs.

After all, we each walk this world differently.

FOR THE FIRST SEVERAL months of #healtheleg, I could still picture what it was like to be active. I could still remember what it felt like to move my body without too much pain. But every day that I woke up with swelling widened the space between the me I knew and missed and the me living in a body I didn't want to be in. Eventually, that space became so big that I couldn't recall any longer what it felt like to wake up, put on my leg and seize the day without a second thought.

I am constantly talking about not letting the things you can't control take control of you and your life, but this one really got me. The constant stop–start of being in pain and discomfort wore me down. Over the past few years, I've done everything I possibly can to try to fix what's going wrong (no jokes — one day I even put cabbage on my foot because someone said that can help reduce swelling), but my body's just not budging. What it does and doesn't do is almost completely out of my control. I know that means I need to focus on what I can control, so that's what I try to do. I can choose how I respond to the situation I'm in, I can choose to concentrate on my mental health, and I can choose to put time and energy into my personal relationships and work life. There's a lot that I can do.

It's not easy. Not at all. I'm not usually a dramatic person, but honestly a lot of the time I feel like I'm partly drowning in waves. Sometimes they're gentle enough that I am able to roll over the top of them and have time to catch my breath, but at other times it's as if I'm in the middle of a storm out at sea. The waves are unexpected and never-ending. But no matter how tempestuous it gets, I try to keep my mind on all of the things I have a say in.

I don't always get it right. There are days — sometimes weeks — where I just sit on the couch feeling angry and frustrated with what I am going through, but I do my best to move on. I'm not going to unpack and live there. And sometimes, right in the thick of it, I might get an intense burst of clarity. I'll realise that there might be other people out there who need to hear about the challenges I'm facing, because that might give them comfort while facing theirs. That's when I might post something like this caption, which I wrote on a particularly bad day in the middle of 2019:

Today I woke up with peak frustration at the current injured state of my leg and then I came across this photo: the first day I got my prosthetic leg.

Imagine being a nine-year-old kid and feeling nothing but excitement for the new leg you're

about to get. I felt invincible. I felt like I was about
to go back to all the things I once knew. Little did
I know that it was going to be a forever project
in learning how to physically do all the things
I wanted to be able to do.

Which made me realise that the only reason
I keep having setbacks is because I've managed
to hold on to that invincibility I had as a kid by
setting myself massive goals (like trying to run
ten kilometres) and doing the things I begin
to doubt I can do (hello, dancing). So I had a
moment today (after serious frustration) when
I realised that that little kid trying on her leg
for the first time would be mind-blown by the
abilities I've gained.

The setbacks are only setbacks in comparison
to all the things I've been able to do. But if I look
from the eyes of that nine-year-old kid, even the
setbacks are nothing but serious achievements.

Perspective. It's a beautiful thing.

ONE DAY RECENTLY, WHEN I was feeling fed up with
the pain in my good leg and the swelling in my other leg, I
said to Mum, 'My groin is so sore. It just won't go away, and
I can't stop it flaring up.'

'I can't wait for you to catch a break soon,' she said. 'For things to all calm down.'

I just sighed and said, 'Honestly, Deb, I don't think that's going to happen in my life. I think this is just the way it goes for me. The thing I really need a break from is the biggest part of my life.'

I instantly felt terrible. I knew it would break her heart to hear me say that, especially when she was being so supportive and sympathetic. No one wants their kid to struggle, ever.

But Mum didn't say anything. She just smiled gently at me.

And that's when I realised she already knew it was true.

After everything I've been through, I've reached an age where I have come to terms with the fact that this life I lead is really hard. There are constant battles. I face challenges every minute of every day — so many that I don't have either the time or the words to even begin to explain them here. Sure, I battled cancer and I lost a leg, but the reality is that one horrific year was actually the easy part. As time passes, things don't necessarily get any easier for me and my body — and I don't actually know if they ever will. For a while, I lived in a bubble where I began to believe that things actually were getting easier, but that bubble has been well and truly popped. This could just be a really long rough patch, or it might simply be what living in this unique body means for me as I get older.

I feel overwhelmed with emotion as I write about all of this, because somewhere in this period that has often felt a lot like hell — the pain, the frustration, the hard reckonings with my reality and my body — I've also been living my life. And, while it's been so tough, it's also been absolutely incredible. I've achieved more than I ever thought possible in the past few years, and I did it all while facing enormous adversity. I wanted to give up so many times, but I didn't. I persevered, and I survived. For that, I'm so proud of myself.

These past few years have taught me that I'm built for this.

It might not be easy, but I'm up for the challenge.

10

Season of stability

They say life is short, but I tend to disagree. Yes, it moves quickly, but life is a marathon.

Maybe my perspective is a little different from the average. The way I see it, life is hard work. You'll need to persevere, and you won't always know quite how you're going to reach the finish line. But, if you're lucky, you won't reach it for a long, long time yet.

So, through the hardship, remember to enjoy the run. Live the life you've been given, even when it's so hard you think it might break you, because I promise you it won't.

Just like me, you will survive. You are strong enough for anything this world throws at you.

BY MARCH 2020, I'D been living in LA for four months. I had a car, I had an apartment, I was modelling, but it wasn't the life in LA I had dreamt of.

On previous work trips, I had spent my nights in the city partying and my days exploring. Now that I lived there, though, I was spending my days trying to get through my work commitments and my nights searching for someone who could help me manage the pain I was in. Every morning I would get up and head to work, carrying my different legs from fittings to castings to photo shoots, and in the evening I would head back to my apartment, remove my leg and — nine times out of ten — cry. It wasn't what I'd pictured living overseas in my twenties would look like. Not at all.

Ever since ruling out medical causes for the swelling in my right leg, I'd been toying with the idea that the problem might be my prosthetic. Maybe it wasn't supporting me correctly any more? Maybe it was time to get a new one designed and built? Sometimes people get a bit confused when I start talking about this, as they assume I've had the exact same prosthetic since I first lost my leg. That's not the case. It's constantly changing as I add different parts. A few times I've had a whole new leg built, but it's always been built in the same way in terms of how it supports me and how it's angled to meet the rest of my body. Maybe it was time for that to change?

I just didn't know where exactly to start looking. What had been difficult to navigate at home was even harder in LA because I was completely on my own. I didn't have my usual support system — not my family, not my physios. I didn't have medical insurance and that meant I simply couldn't receive the kind of treatment I got at home, the treatment I needed to get through the day. One thing I did have, though, was easier access to a wider set of experts than I'd had back at home. In New Zealand, there are just a handful of us with a rotationplasty, so that means services are naturally limited, but the numbers and the expertise increase in proportion to the population here in the States.

Another thing I had was the incredible community of people from all over the world who had signed up to hear the parts of my story I chose to share on Instagram. So, on one especially tearful, helpless night, I decided to put the question to them.

'Does anyone know of an amazing prosthetist or company in the USA who has worked with rotationplasty amputees?' I asked.

I figured it was unlikely I'd get the same torrent of responses as I would if I'd asked for the best coffee in town, but I was pleasantly surprised when the recommendations came pouring in.

Every amputee gave the same reply: 'Hanger Clinic.'

I googled the name and learnt that Hanger Clinic is a prosthetics leg, arm and hand provider with clinics across the States. I immediately emailed them to ask who their best rotationplasty prosthetist was. 'I'm happy to travel anywhere in the USA,' I wrote, although by this point I was so desperate it would have been more accurate to say I would have travelled to Mars if that's what was required. They replied the next day, putting me in touch with a guy called Monte in San Diego, which is just a three-hour drive from LA. Monte wrote to say he'd worked with other rotationplasty amputees who had dealt with swelling, and that one guy in particular had gone through something similar to my experience over the past few years.

And just like that, I felt an enormous sense of relief. I wasn't alone in what I was going through any more. Finally, someone had heard me and understood me.

I might have even found the person who could help me.

THE NEXT DAY, I jumped on a video call with Monte to learn a bit more about what he could offer.

I was mindful not to get my hopes up too much, because I'd already talked to so many professionals who hadn't been able to help me. This time, though, the main difference was that, while no one else had ever even heard of someone with a rotationplasty, Monte had a whole lot of experience working with people like me — and, as I was about to discover, his connection with his clients was even more personal than I could have possibly imagined. Not only had Monte made prosthetics for hundreds of people with a rotationplasty, but he had also battled a similar cancer to me back in 2003 — just two years after I did, but he was older than I had been. He also lost his leg. He also had a rotationplasty. And that guy he'd referred to with the swelling similar to mine? That was *him*.

Not only was Monte a professional expert in rotation-plasty amputations, he was also a personal expert.

I got off that call and felt so relieved I cried. I'd finally met someone who had walked a similar path to mine. I was filled with hope that if anyone could help me, it would be Monte.

MONTE'S PLAN WAS TO build me a new prosthetic from scratch. He said it would take three days from start to finish (which blew my mind when I thought about the months it had taken to get my blade built) and I would need to come down to San Diego.

By that time, I'd reached the end of my tether with living in LA. My swollen leg wasn't getting any better, and I'd decided it was time to put my body first. I had a work commitment back in New Zealand at the start of March, so I'd organised to move back home at the same time, with the plan being that I would head over to LA every few months for work as necessary.

The only three days that I could be in San Diego happened to be my last three days in the States. Since I didn't have insurance, I had to fund the prosthetic myself. It was going to cost upwards of US$10,000, but I didn't care about that right then — I put it on a payment plan and locked in the dates with Monte. It was a massive financial risk to take. A leg isn't exactly the kind of thing you can return with proof of purchase for a refund, but my gut was telling me this was the way to go. I had originally planned to stay in San Diego for those three days, but I ended up needing to be in LA to sort out some last bits and pieces before moving home, so I decided to do three day trips in a row. I knew I was mad, but I had to find a way to make it work.

Meeting Monte in person for the first time was amazing. It was actually kind of confronting to find myself face to face with someone who had the same amputation as me. It might sound a bit strange, but as familiar as I was with my own leg, I'd only ever looked down on it. Seeing someone else with a rotationplasty made me suddenly think, *Oh wow, I have the same thing. I guess this is sort of what other people see when they look at me.* I had a million questions I wanted to ask him, but as we were pushed for time I kept it to what was necessary (although I did manage to slip in the odd question about his experience growing up in a body like ours).

Meeting Monte in person for the first time was amazing. It was actually kind of confronting to find myself face to face with someone who had the same amputation as me.

After reviewing my current leg, Monte explained how he was going to do things differently for my new leg. It would look the same as the old leg from the outside, but on the inside everything — from the angle my foot sat on to the socket and the way the joint would move and support me — would be different. For me, the change was going to be huge. As I've mentioned, each time I make even a minor adjustment to my prosthetic, it takes my body a long time to adapt. Getting a whole new leg made in a completely different way? I would essentially be learning to walk again.

I drove three hours back to LA that evening filled with so much hope, and the next morning I got back in my car and drove all the way back again for my first fitting. As I expected, everything was completely foreign: the way this new leg felt against my skin, the way my foot sat so snugly in the corset, even the feeling of the different sock I was wearing within the socket. I was instantly transported back to being that hopeful nine-year-old trying on her new leg for the first time. All these years later, the experience was the same — I went from *I have a new leg!* to *I have a new leg . . . Now I need to learn to walk with it.* And just like back then, I knew I had no other choice but to stick with it if I wanted the best chance at getting back the life I once had. The only difference, of course, is that as a kid I was trying to get back my life with two legs, whereas now I was trying to get back to the life I'd found with my prosthetic.

The next morning, when I drove back to San Diego one last time, my flight home to New Zealand was only 48 hours away. What if my leg wasn't ready? What if I wasn't ready? I wished I could spend a month with Monte, making sure the leg was exactly right, but I simply didn't have that kind of time. I reassured myself by remembering that I would be back in a month or two — I could rehab at home, then come back to him for adjustments and answers to the flood of questions I was sure to have.

That last day was the hardest of all. The whole leg was

done and ready for me to put on. Everything felt more foreign than ever. The corset was now made of plastic, not leather, and was uncomfortable. The socket was tighter than my old prosthetic, and at first that made no sense because the issue I was having was swelling — the last thing I wanted was something tighter. At one point, Monte left the room to make a couple of adjustments, and I started crying. I felt so overwhelmed. Here I was, on my own, trying to navigate a huge change and wondering whether I'd just made a massive mistake. I felt alone. I felt scared. And I felt frustrated when I thought about how long the road ahead was going to be. I knew how much time it was going to take for me to get familiar with this new leg. Fortunately, this was a feeling I'd got used to — the sense of uncertainty right before something big happened — so I sat with it, and by the time Monte returned I'd put my smiley face back on. I knew it was at least worth a try.

Here I was, on my own, trying to navigate a huge change and wondering whether I'd just made a massive mistake.

Monte explained that the socket needed to be tight to stop my foot constantly pulling out as I walked. When I took my first ungainly step, I felt so unstable. Since my foot was still swollen, it was hard to make adjustments. I didn't know whether things were hurting because the leg wasn't fitting right or because of the swelling. I walked up and down the room, trying to make sure everything was as it should be. We made as many adjustments as possible, and eventually reached a place where everything felt good. My three days with Monte were up — and this was huge. Usually with a new prosthetic, I'd have the chance over those first few months to go into a clinic regularly and make all of the little adjustments that came up as I learnt to walk with my new leg, but I wasn't going to be able to do that with Monte. I wouldn't see him until I came back to LA.

Monte cautioned me not to wear my new leg on the way back home, so I headed back to New Zealand with it packed safely in my suitcase. I spent my first week back home in bed — my leg had swollen up so badly on the flight home that, even if I could get my prosthetic on, I couldn't put any weight through it. I couldn't wear my new leg, let alone start practising walking with it. I had to wait for the swelling to go down first, so I was back to what had become my normal practice of ice, legs up the wall and rest.

But, just as things began to settle for me and I started thinking about getting back into my life at home, the whole world changed. Covid-19 went from something we'd been hearing about on the news to something that stopped us all in our tracks. At one minute before midnight on 25 March 2020, New Zealand shut its borders and went into a nationwide lockdown. We were confined to the four walls of our homes, except for when we ventured outside — and even then we had to stay at least two metres from anyone we passed.

The realisation hit me then that I would not be going back to LA any time soon. Who knew when I would get to see Monte in person again?

I was on my own once more, this time learning to walk with my new leg.

THE STORY OF MY rehabilitation into my new leg is so long it could fill a whole other book.

It ended up taking me a long time to muster the strength to even put my leg on. It sat packaged up in my wardrobe throughout our first six-week-long lockdown. It's hard to explain why, but I think there's a mental process I have to go through when I get a new leg. It's like I have to come to terms with the change before I can allow it to fully happen.

There was also the aesthetic side of it. My previous prosthetic had looked like a leg in every way possible. It had a skin on it that matched the skin on my good leg. It had toes and veins, and a foot that was shaped just like a real foot. I'd got it six years earlier, once I stopped growing, and I loved it. I loved the way I could look down and see ten toes. I was so attached to this leg and its skin, but I also knew the time had come for change. My new leg didn't have the same skin. Letting go of my old leg meant letting go of having its skin. And, actually, I was surprised by how okay I was with that in the end. As well as physically outgrowing that leg over six years, I'd also had enough time to grow emotionally, to a point where I didn't need my leg to look exactly like a leg any more. Sure, some days I do still wish I had toes and could wear the shoes I wore with my old leg, given the shape of its foot, but I've reached a place in my life where function is so much more important than form. A leg that looks like a leg is nice, but a leg that works like a leg is better.

When it comes to learning to actually walk with my new leg, though, let me just say it's been a complicated, tiresome and frustrating process, where I go from wondering whether things don't feel right just because they're new, or because they are, in fact, not right. One year and three lockdowns later, I'm sitting here wearing my new leg as I write, but the world still hasn't opened up again. I still can't go back to LA to check in with Monte. Being able to jump on a plane to visit him would have made this whole process so much easier. It's hard to express just how much one-on-one time usually goes into fine-tuning a prosthetic. Once you get it made and you've had a chance to wear it, you'll then go in for regular check-ups to ensure everything is still correctly aligned as your body adapts. I haven't had that, because I haven't been able to go and see Monte. We've spoken over video a handful of times, and he keeps reassuring me that I'm on the right track. 'It's just a slow process,' he says.

Slow doesn't really cover it. Only in the last few weeks have I been able to walk further than a few hundred metres. For a long time, even a lap around the supermarket was enough to force me to stop and sit down out of discomfort. Over the past few months, though, the discomfort has shifted from being about having a foot so swollen I can't walk, to being solely about learning to navigate wearing a foreign prosthetic. I have had only a handful of swollen days during this time, and even on those days it hasn't been bad enough to send me back to bed.

Slow doesn't really cover it. Only in the last few weeks have I been able to walk further than a few hundred metres. For a long time, even a lap around the supermarket was enough to force me to stop and sit down out of discomfort.

I'm cautious to not get too excited, but I'm finally starting to feel like maybe, after two long years, things might be coming right. My right foot no longer looks like it's been stung by a bee when I remove my prosthetic at night, and I'm gradually beginning to remember what it feels like to wake up in the morning without wondering whether or not my leg is going to go on. I'm starting to feel what it might be like to get my abilities back. I can't even begin to express how enormous it is to write that last sentence. As I reread it now, I feel like I can take a big, deep breath for the first time in a very long time.

Sometimes, it feels like I don't have space left for anything besides surviving, and even that can feel overwhelming. It's a lot. But the good news is that, even though it's still challenging, I do feel like I'm finally starting to get my stride back.

As for my left leg? The injury in my groin on that side is still present. It's not 100 per cent yet, but things are starting to look up. I go to physio every day, and am doing intense rehab and receiving all sorts of treatment to try to get things right. On top of this, my whole body is wound tight as a spring as a result of working so hard to compensate for the pain I've been suffering all this time. And then there's the toll that everything about the past two years — the pain, the discomfort, the uncertainty and the unanswered questions — has taken on my mental health, to the point that I'm now getting professional help for that too. It's like my tolerance for anything has been totally obliterated, and I have days where even holding a conversation or trying to enjoy the good times feels impossible. Sometimes, it feels like I don't have space left for anything besides surviving, and even that can feel overwhelming. It's a lot. But the good news is that, even though it's still challenging, I do feel like I'm finally starting to get my stride back.

It's fair to say that the road ahead is long. It's also fair to say it might stretch on past the horizon. Who knows?

If I've learnt anything over the past two years, it's the importance of putting my body first. For a while, I think I felt incapable if I wasn't pushing myself beyond the limits of what should have been physically possible, but something in me has changed. Maybe I'm just growing up, but I've begun to understand that the price of pushing myself so hard might be years afterwards of trying to regain a life without pain. I'll forever be chasing some kind of goal, but I've well and truly proved to myself that I can achieve things that seem impossible — or, at the very least, give them everything I've got so I always know I've tried my hardest. What matters most to me now is being able to live my life doing the day-to-day activities that make it richer. I've redefined what I want to be able to do. I want to live in a body that doesn't hurt. I want to go for a walk with my sister, Abby, and her daughter, Zadie, my niece, who was born in 2020. I want to take one of the Pilates classes Soph's started teaching since becoming an instructor. I want to go on adventures at the weekend with my partner and puppy.

I want to wake up and not wonder, *What's going to hold me back today?*

I feel like I am entering a new season of my life. I no longer need to prove things to myself. I know what I'm capable of, and I know it's much more than that little girl lying in her hospital bed could ever have imagined. But I also know I didn't fight so hard for this life in order to be constantly testing its limits.

Now, I want to be able to live the life I fought for without needing to prove things to myself, without the pain.

Here's to this new season. The season of stability.

PRETTY MUCH EVERY TIME I do an interview, people will hear about all the things I've faced in this life and say, 'Wow, you have so much strength,' or, 'I can't imagine getting through that.'

It always gets me thinking. I genuinely believe we are all stronger than we know. It's just that it usually takes life putting us to the test for us to know our own strength. And, as I look back over 2020, I realise it was the sort of year that probably taught all of us that lesson. At the end of the year, a memory popped up on my Instagram of a post I'd made on the same day in 2019. 'No matter what this next year brings,' I had written, 'know that you have the strength within you to handle anything this life throws at you.' I was writing that having just survived what had been one of the most personally difficult years of my life. I had no idea just how many people were going to need messages like that in the year to come.

At the start of 2020, none of us could have predicted what the year would bring, but I think it's safe to say it's a year we will never forget. We were all challenged more than ever, in more ways than one. As I've said, adversity isn't biased. No amount of money, fame or success can save you from the unthinkable — but I believe a lot of us, so long as hardship doesn't really touch us, hope we might somehow escape the inevitable. We tell ourselves the bad things won't happen to us. Bad things happen only to others. Except that's obviously not true. Hardship can come for any of us, at any time, and 2020 reminded us all of that truth.

I don't say this to scare you. I don't say it so that you live your life in constant fear that terrible things will happen. I say it to remind you that when you see someone else facing hard times, they are no different from me or you. I say it to remind you to never, ever take your life for granted, because at any given moment the unexpected could happen. I say it to remind you that you don't have to wait for the worst to happen to learn just how strong you are. Please trust me on this.

I have been through challenges that have taught me that I am stronger than anything that tries to break me in this life.

So are you.

I have learnt that I am stronger than the battles I face.

So are you.

> **I knew I had a choice. I could live a
> life of misery because of the things that
> had happened to me or I could live
> a life of happiness regardless of the
> things that had happened to me.**

Strength is something that lives within all of us, but we have to choose to see it. People always ask me 'Where did you get your strength?' and, honestly, I just never saw the point in living any other way. I knew I had a choice. I could live a life of misery because of the things that had happened to me or I could live a life of happiness regardless of the things that had happened to me. I just knew that if I focused on all the ways my life was hard it would only become harder. But if I focused on the positives, the things I could control? Then I knew I would be able to live my best life. That choice was mine. It's the same choice we all have. You only get this one life. Why not do everything you can to make it amazing?

I'm also not the only one who has been strong — so have my parents, my sisters and everyone who loves me. Adversity isn't an island. It doesn't just affect one of us at a time. I can't even express how much I have my mum, dad and sisters to thank for their strength. They led by example. They knew that they had to be strong in order to get me through. They helped me see the positives when it felt like there were none. They gave me so much to fight for. So I guess my strength came from two places: there was the fire I had within me to push on, but it also came from my family.

A while ago, I was digging through some old photos and among them I found what looked like a letter. I unfolded it and saw my mum's handwriting scribbled across a few pages. It was notes for a speech she gave to my class at school just three days before my leg was amputated. I went to a small school, and my friends had all sent me letters and photos while I was going through chemo to keep me up to date with everything. They'd even fundraised for me to get a TV in my bedroom at home. They were like family. They were feeling the effects of what I was going through too. So imagine going and standing in front of them, a room full of eight-year-olds with bright and expectant eyes all fixed on you, and explaining calmly and carefully exactly what was going to happen to your little girl, their friend.

Well, that's exactly what my mum did. Her strength has blown me away so many times, but knowing she'd done this was something else. I'm sure she wished I was just one of those kids sitting on the classroom floor. I'm sure she wished she didn't have to be strong right then, but she was. She gave that speech.

She'd called it 'Jessica's Journey', and in a little box in the margin she'd written down what must have been some notes to herself. Among them was one that read, 'Write a book together.' Even back then, she had thought I should share my story — and here I am, exactly 20 years later, doing just that, in ways she could never have dreamt of while I was still stuck in that hospital.

First, she explained to my classmates why I wasn't there with them that day. She talked about the tumour — 'a group of troublesome cells' — in my femur, then she told them about 'Captain Chemo', which was 'leading an army going into war and killing off as much of the badness as it can'. Then she told them what was going to happen to my leg:

> Jessica has a great doctor who found out about
> an amazing but unusual operation that some
> American children have had but not many
> in New Zealand have. This is a very special
> operation. It will be quite hard at first to imagine
> how Jess's new leg will look, but on Thursday her
> doctor is going to remove her thigh and use the
> good part of her leg, which is below the knee,
> including her foot, then turn the leg around and
> attach it to Jessica's hip. This means that her lower
> calf will be her thigh and her backwards foot will
> be her knee. But what about the lower bit? What

will Jessica's leg look like? Without a doubt, her leg will look very odd.

Jessica will get a new special leg called a prosthesis. It will be specially made for her. Every time she gets up in the morning, she will need to put her new leg on and then her shoes. We might have to get up a lot earlier every morning!

The excellent news is she will be able to walk and even do some sports without crutches — and, boy, Jess will love to throw those crutches away. She gets sore hands!

Jessica will need lots of letters and emails. She is going to need your support and understanding for some time. Thanks to you and your families for all of your wonderful support this year.

Ah, Mum. You will forever amaze me. People ask me where my strength comes from. I think this says it all. (Oh, and Mum, I wrote that book.)

IN 2020, PEOPLE ALL over the world found themselves physically separated from one other, and that actually seemed to bring us closer than ever. For the first time, many of us realised that we were all, truly, in this together. Before Covid-19, we might have heard of people or countries or cities facing hardship elsewhere and felt sad about it, but it didn't really affect us. We moved on quickly. The global pandemic has affected all of us, every single one, regardless of our differences.

We have learnt that we have this one thing in common: we are all climbing our own mountains. We all struggle along the way. Some of us reach our summits, while others have to find another way round. It might not always be possible to see what someone else is dealing with. Their scars might be hidden. Their battles might be happening behind closed doors or determined smiles.

Just know that every single human you encounter has a story to tell. Every single human has something they wish never happened or a fear they hope will never eventuate. Every single human has dreams they barely dare to believe possible.

We need to support one another on this journey. We need to be kind to one another. And we need to be kind to ourselves. So ask yourself each morning, 'How can I be kinder today?' Remind yourself that the person who just swerved in front of you in traffic might be struggling to stay afloat in the waves battering them. That the cashier at the supermarket who didn't smile back at you might be living through a world of pain. That the parent with their baby trying to lift a pushchair onto the bus could do with a hand.

No matter what, be kind. Do it without expecting

anything in return. The world won't always be kind to you, but that doesn't mean you shouldn't be kind.

Remember that you are unique. You are different, but being different is the one thing we all have in common.

Beauty exists within us all, and it comes in many forms. Don't get caught in the trap of believing there's only one narrow view of beauty.

There is no wrong way to have a body, so wear the shorts, live a life you're proud of and don't hide your insecurities. We all have them. Live a life *because* of your body, not in spite of it.

This life is hard, but it is also incredible. Quite clearly mine isn't perfect — not even close — but life doesn't have to be perfect to be amazing. After all, you can't live a life and not allow life to happen to you. That means being there for the ups and the downs.

If I could tell my younger self anything, it would be this:

Let people in.

Don't push love or affection away.

Know your body is made to take you places, not to be picked apart.

Remember that you are a match for your mountains. Trust that you have the strength that you need inside you. All you have to do is use it.

Allow yourself to be soft while remaining strong. You can be both. Please, be both.

Let the people who knock in. Let them help you. Let them love you. You don't have to do it all on your own.

It's not going to be easy. In fact, it will be harder than you can imagine, but it becomes more worth it with every day you live.

Remember that whenever it feels like it won't get better, it will. Every time. Trust me.

You have everything you need within you to live your best life.

You've got this.

Acknowledgements

OUT OF ALL THE pages in this book, these ones have been the hardest to write. Okay, that may be a slight exaggeration, but where I start and where I stop has been weighing on my mind for weeks. Given the life I have lived up until this point, the list of people who have made me who I am — who have supported me, cheered me on and helped build me back up — is endless.

First and foremost, I want to thank you, the reader. The fact that this book is currently in your hands and you've just read it (unless you skipped straight to the acknowledgements to see if you are in here) is mind-blowing to me. I have wanted to write a book since I was a nine-year-old girl lying in bed without my newly amputated right leg, but I could never have imagined that dream would turn into this. Over the years I've spent writing, I have always had a ping of self-doubt in my head: *Will anyone actually want to read this?* The fact that it's in your hands is proof that someone did, and that makes me want to do a happy dance. After all, this book is for you: the you that feels 'different', the you that has faced hardship after hardship, the you that has at some point hidden away because of your insecurities. Thank you, and I hope you see that hope always has a place in this world.

To Jenny and the team at Allen & Unwin, thank you

for seeing something in me and inviting me to become an author. You have made one of my biggest dreams come true and for that I will be forever grateful.

To Kimberley Davis, who patiently moulded my words into something that makes me so proud. Thank you for believing in my story and helping me get it out to the world. Thank you for teaching me everything I now know about book writing. As I've told you many times over, I am in awe of your talent, your hard work and your ability to turn my often jumbled thoughts and words into something worth reading.

To Brooke Howard-Smith, thank you for constantly pushing me to do the things that scare me most. Thank you for seeing my potential and helping me achieve wild things.

To the brands that have backed me on this adventure and the many other adventures I have had, thank you. The fact that you stand by my message means the world to me. A huge thank you to the team at AIA (I have been an AIA Vitality ambassador since May 2019). Your dedication to helping people is something I respect and admire, and I am so grateful for you all.

Seriously, I wasn't kidding when I said I have so many people to thank — from those who have been involved in my writing journey right back to those who have supported me and my family from 2001 and onwards. I need to thank every healthcare worker I have been lucky enough to cross paths with. The nurses, the doctors, the anaesthetist, the physios, the chiropractors, the radiologists and so many more. I often look back on the years that I spent going in and out of hospital and smile. That might sound weird, given how many traumatic things I experienced, but what sticks with me are the people who helped me. I am forever grateful to those who helped paint the bad memories with a bit of colour. And to every healthcare worker who has helped me on my rehab journey since, thank you.

To Mike Hanlon, thank you for thinking outside the box and giving me the life I have now. Rotationplasty was a scary option back in 2001, but I hope you know, through the life I have lived, that everything I can do today is because of you.

To every single friend I have had over the years through to this moment, thank you for never making me feel different and for supporting me when I needed it.

I am one of those lucky humans with many aunties, uncles and cousins who are like second parents and siblings. We may be a loud family, but the love we all have for each other makes me so happy. And, to Mary-Rose, who is also an aunty to me, I can never thank you enough for the ways in which you so selflessly show up for me and my family. I love my extended family so much.

To Grandma Ann, your love for books has been an inspiration for mine. I still remember you sitting by my hospital bed when I was sick and making me laugh. I have so many fond memories of 'dates with Nanny' and delicious mac and cheese — I am so lucky to have a gran like you, and I love you so very much.

To Nana Jan, who I lost while writing this book. I still have to remind myself that you're not here and it hurts every time. I know you would be parading this book around all of your friends, just like you did with everything I ever achieved. I will love you forever.

I was 26 when I embarked on writing this book and, honestly, even though I was still young, I was beginning to wonder if I would ever find a love like the one I have witnessed throughout my life between my parents. Then, halfway through writing this book, Todd showed up in my life and changed that completely. Todd, you've very quickly become my best friend and partner in crime. You entered my life at my most turbulent time and have continued to love and support me without question. Apologies for the nights I kept you up wondering if I should write more or start the whole book again. I am one lucky girl to have you by my side.

And, finally, to my whole reason for being: my family. Mum, Dad, Abby and Sophie-Rose, there aren't enough words in the English language to describe my love for you.

To Abby and Sophie-Rose, you two are the best friends I could ever have asked for. I'm sorry you had to go through all that when we were so young, and I'm sorry I took so much of Mum and Dad's attention away from you, but I am beyond grateful for the ways in which you supported me then and every day since. You two are the most selfless humans I know, and I idolise you both every day. Thank you for always giving me the front seat without putting up a fight, thank you for the never-ending belly laughs and for never treating me any different, and thank you for always being just a phone call away.

To Mum and Dad — wow, I have a lump in my throat just thinking about how much I love you. It's also kind of hilarious how many random strangers will be reading this, but hey, this life I live can be strange sometimes. Writing this book opened my eyes to just how much you both went through when I was a girl. Thank you for making the hard decisions when I couldn't — I hope the life I have lived shows you that you made the right call. Thank you for not wrapping me in cotton wool and for giving me the opportunity to figure this new life out on my own, and thank you for always being there when I took that a little too far. You are the reason I so fearlessly go after everything I want in life, and it's because you never made me believe I couldn't. My biggest thank you goes to both of you — and this is something we three girls always talk about — for the way you endlessly love each other (and us). It's been a privilege to grow up seeing and feeling a love like that.

They say you can't pick your family but, honestly, I'd pick you four time and time again.

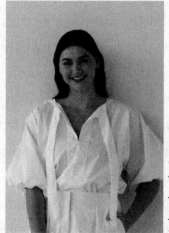

Author photo by Brijana Cato

About the author

JESS QUINN is an advocate for normalising 'different'. She champions this through her social media platform, her speaking engagements and her role as a brand ambassador.